my soul waits

# my soul waits

finding hope through miscarriage

Michelle Ng

ISBN: 978-0-646-81277-9

Independently published.

Printed in Melbourne, Australia by Ingram Spark

Cover photo and design by: Jonathan Ng

Dedicated to Jonathan, my love.
I'm so grateful for who you are, and for who I am because of you.

I wait on the Lord, my soul waits, and in his word I put my hope
(Psalm130:5)

This book is for my dear friends and women everywhere, who have lost a baby during pregnancy or childbirth.

It's for the mums and dads who left the hospital without their precious babe in their arms; those who would give anything to hold their child against their chest, just once, or one more time.

It's for those who walk amongst us with heavy hearts, those whose world fell out from underneath you, when you were told your baby's heart had stopped beating.

This book is for all of us who think about our babies every single day, and who will always wonder what could have been.

It's for anyone who has ever wondered, am I brave enough, strong enough, courageous enough, to go on without my baby?

All of our experiences are different, but your pain is warranted, your grief is real and you are not alone. Even in the darkest of valleys we can find hope and strength to keep moving forward.

Beautiful mumma, I hope this book reveals to you that there is something inside of you that is stronger than you could ever imagine, and you are more than enough. For every day you've survived since losing your precious child, you are amazing.

My babies' names are Preston, Gabriel, Raphie and Theodore. This is our story.

# 1

## preston

The fluro lights pierced my eyes as I woke up in the recovery unit, dazed and confused. I could hear a machine beeping to the left of me and the nurse shuffling between each bed. As my eyes began to focus I remembered where I was and what had happened. The nurse moved in close to check my vital signs and I grabbed her hand.

"Where's my baby?" I asked her. "Is my baby ok?"

"I wasn't told my dear," the nurse said. "It's just my job to look after you, try to rest for now ok."

Rest? How could I rest? My eyes darted around the room, desperately looking for somebody who could give me some answers.

I thought back on the day's events and my heart started to ache.

It had only been a few hours since I left work on that sunny Friday morning. I was 34 weeks pregnant, and decided to go to the hospital because I couldn't feel my baby moving.

My husband Jonathan was at home renovating our house. I contemplated driving home to have lunch with him on the way, but when I reached the intersection that would lead to our house or the

3

hospital, I had this overwhelming sense of urgency to go straight to the hospital.

I'm glad I did. Preston was delivered by an emergency c-section within 15 minutes of my arrival. There was no time to wait for Jonathan to be there, not even enough time for an epidural. They gave me a general anaesthetic so they could deliver the baby straight away.

Things happened so quickly. As they prepped me for surgery the nurse told me that if there was something wrong with my baby's heart that he or she might be at another hospital by the time I woke up. I tried to hold my peace.

Just before I went to sleep I glanced to the corner of the room and saw the nurses from the special care unit. They were standing by a small bed with oxygen on hand and a heat lamp, ready to take care of my baby. I said a quick prayer for them and slowly counted backwards from 10…

When I woke from my surgery I was dazed and desperate for answers. "Is my baby ok?" I asked every nurse and doctor who walked by. Nobody could answer me.

The anaesthetist from my surgery came in with another patient, and as our eyes met I think he could see my heartache. He came over to my bedside and took my hand. "Is the baby ok?" I asked, holding in my tears. He squeezed my hand tight. "Everything went well," he said. "It's ok."

Not really a straight answer, but it gave me hope. I closed my eyes and tried not to cry. The nurse from the ward came in to take me to my room. "Boy or girl?" she asked. "I have no idea." I answered. "Can you please find out if my baby is ok?"

She had a quick look at my file and started unlocking the brakes on my bed. "Let's go and find your baby," she said.

I took a deep breath.

Jonathan met us in the hallway as they wheeled me down the corridor. It was so good to see him. I knew he would have the answers. His camera strap was hanging over his shoulder and the smile on his face filled my heart with joy.

He took my hand. Tears filled my eyes and I felt my heart jump into my throat.

"Is the baby ok?" I cried.

"Yes," he said.

"Boy or girl?" I asked.

"A boy!".

I'll never forget the smile on Jonathan's face when he told me it was a boy. My heart ached to see my baby, but I was so glad that his dad was with him when I couldn't be.

We turned the corner and entered the special care nursery. I was still recovering from the general anaesthetic, but the desire to see my baby was much stronger than my desire to go back to sleep. It had been a long, exhausting and traumatic day, but my heart was so desperate to see him. I needed to hold my baby. I needed to see for myself that he was ok. I needed to touch his skin and kiss his forehead. I needed him to know that I was there.

The nurse wheeled me in and parked my bed next to his. I looked into the humidicrib to see the most beautiful, tiny, dark-haired, baby boy staring back at me.

For a moment time stood still. I could hear Jonathan's camera clicking away in the background. There were doctors and nurses talking to each other, asking questions and writing notes. Across the room other premature babies were laying in their cribs sleeping and growing.

So much was happening in every direction, but to me it was all white noise. All that mattered was my little baby laying across from me. I felt a tear run down the side of my face. I couldn't believe what had just happened. I couldn't believe he was here.

He was four hours old the first time I looked into the eyes of my sweet baby boy. I wasn't the beginning I had hoped for, but still a precious moment for us both. The nurse took Preston out of the humidicrib and placed him underneath my hospital gown. The side of his head was resting on my chest, listening to the familiar sound of my heart beat. He fed for a while and then snuggled back into my chest again.

My baby was here. Six weeks early, but he was here. He had survived a huge blood clot in my umbilical cord. I had no idea how, or why this had happened, but I knew this boy was special and that he was meant to be here. The specialist told me that if I had come to the hospital an hour or two later things would have been very different. Preston would not have survived.

My heart ached for what had been, and it broke for what could have been. But in that moment all that mattered was that I had my baby safe in my arms. The sound of my heartbeat put him back to sleep, and with the rise and fall of his tiny chest, I closed my eyes and fell asleep too.

## 2

<hr/>

# relentless

The days, weeks and months following Preston's birth were so beautiful. I loved being his mum and I loved every minute being at home with my little boy. He was so quiet and content. He hardly ever cried. This tiny human being fit so perfectly into our family, and we were so blessed that he was finally here.

I often wondered what my life would have been like if I didn't go to the hospital that day. How would my heart have coped if the worst had happened? I entered motherhood being told that there was a short two hours between life or death for my baby. The thought of what could have been was always in the back of my mind, and as the physical scars began to heal, the emotional ones came to the surface.

The first few years of his life were literally a whirlwind. A journey of love, hope, faith and healing. Preston was absolutely perfect. He passed every milestone test and had all of the doctors and nurses forgetting that he was born prematurely. He grew into a clever, inquisitive, loving and sensitive little boy, whose chubby cheeks would melt the heart of everyone he met.

Despite how amazing my little boy was, the trauma surrounding his birth had taken its toll on me. I soon felt overcome by an overwhelming sense of protection and subsequent anxiety that would follow for the next few years.

After Preston turned one, I became really sick. I suffered with severe stomach pain and vomiting episodes that would have me on the bathroom floor anywhere from six, to thirty-six hours, and this re-occurred every two to three weeks. This continued for about twelve months. It was relentless.

We knew that having another baby was out of the question while I was so sick. Who knows what harm it could do to the baby while I was pregnant, and I struggled enough to take care of one child while I was so sick let alone two.

I had every medical test possible, but got no answers. Following the advice of my doctor I turned to a psychologist for help. She helped me through some issues including the separation anxiety that I had suffered throughout my childhood, the trauma of Preston's birth, and the subsequent fear I had trusting anyone else to look after him. I also had some prayer ministry sessions with my pastor and the elders at my church.

Over time, the frequency of the vomiting slowed down and it eventually stopped. When Preston turned two, my health was in a much better state. We decided that after Christmas we would start trying for another baby. We wanted more than anything for Preston to have a little brother or sister to share his life with. We had waited so long for my health to improve, so it was a great blessing that it only took two months for us to fall pregnant.

This is where my next chapter begins.

## 3

---

# the pee stick

I sat on the end of my bed in silence. Preston was in the lounge room watching Paw Patrol and Jonathan was asleep behind me. I looked at the clock. It was time to go back in.

I slowly stood up, but then shook my head and sat back down again. The pregnancy test I had taken just minutes before, was sitting on my bathroom vanity waiting to tell me our fate. I was so excited to see the answer, but at the same time I knew how disappointed I would be if I wasn't pregnant.

I stood up again and slowly walked into the bathroom. As my eyes focused on the result window I saw the two pink lines and instantly I fell in love.

My knees hit the floor as I cried and prayed. It was exactly the same as when I found out I was pregnant with Preston two years before. Both times I knelt down and thanked God that He would trust me with such a precious gift. Both times I asked him to help me to be the best mum I could be, and to give my babies the best future possible, where they would always feel cherished and loved.

I'll never forget those moments. Both so similar yet on two very different bathroom floors. I took the pregnancy test for Preston in our hotel room in Hawaii back in 2014. Two years later I was at home, in our newly renovated bathroom, when I found out baby number two was on the way.

I felt so happy to be pregnant again, overjoyed actually. The love in my heart instantly doubled. I felt a strong connection with my baby and immediately started planning the next nine months in my head.

I was so hopeful for what was to come.

I had no reason to think that anything would go wrong. To me, this baby was the answer to our prayers. We had been through so much with my health and things were finally better. We waited until I was well enough to have a baby, and really felt it was God's perfect timing. I felt like nothing could take the joy from my heart.

That morning I asked Preston to draw me a picture of a baby. When he finished I wrote "Preston's baby" above his drawing and the due date on the back. When Jonathan came out for breakfast Preston gave the picture to him and that's how he found out we were pregnant.

He smiled the exact same smile that he did in our hotel room two years ago, when I told him we we pregnant the first time. A smile of pure joy, excitement and amazement that we were going to have a baby.

This was the missing piece to our puzzle. The beautiful child that would complete our family. My heart was full of love. I felt so blessed and had everything I had ever hoped and dreamed for.

That morning in our living room with my husband, toddler and our new baby safe inside of me, things were perfect. So much love, so much excitement, so much hope for what could be, so much riding on that one little pee stick.

# 4

# early days

It was the first day of my new job. I stood in my wardrobe all morning staring at my clothes. I thought about how long it would take before nothing would fit me again, and I'd have to dig out the maternity bag stuffed in the back of the linen cupboard.

Part of me was excited for the new job. The other part didn't want to leave Preston at home while he was so little. He was growing up so quickly, and I didn't want to miss anything. Being pregnant made going back to work a little easier, because I knew it wasn't forever.

I told them in my job interview that we were trying for a baby. Little did I know we were already pregnant. The job was perfect. I was working two days a week with such lovely people, and felt it was a great balance between work and home life. I didn't tell anyone at the office we were expecting. We had only just met and the morning sickness was under control, so I didn't feel the need to tell anyone just yet.

At home things were different. Preston was so excited when I told him I had a baby in my belly. He would pat my belly and give it kisses and cuddles. Just like his mum and dad, big brother Preston was smitten already. I have a video of Preston standing in our kitchen dancing around yelling "mummy baby in her belly" over and over again. My heart felt so full. He was going to be the most amazing big brother and I couldn't wait.

Our secret seemed safe until one day when Preston and his grandma were having a playdate through a video call. My mum lived four hours away so Preston would often play with his cars in the toy room or playdough at the dining room table with grandma sitting across from him on my phone.

One day I was folding clothes in the next room when Preston stood up and flashed a bit of his stomach at grandma. "Look at your belly" she said, to which Preston replied "Mummy baby in belly!" My mum didn't say a word, and I kept folding as though nothing had happened. She didn't know that I heard what he said and so she kept this secret to herself, waiting for our announcement.

I decided I needed to tell somebody my good news. I found a safe place in my friend Julia from my mothers group. She had been gently encouraging me to have another baby for a while now and I knew she would be so excited. I sent her a photo of the pregnancy test, then I sat staring at my phoning, awaiting her response. It was even better than I expected. So much joy, so much excitement. It was so good to share my news with somebody who I knew would love my baby as much as she loved me. I couldn't wait to tell all of our family and friends that a new baby was on the way.

Aside from a little nausea I was feeling good. Another week went by and I decided to start booking all of our appointments. First ultrasound, first midwife appointment and my blood tests. We were all booked in months ahead and ready to roll.

Jonathan and I also started shopping for a bigger family car and a big boy bed for Preston. We knew that we had plenty of time, but I wanted him to have his bed ready well before the new baby arrived. The renovations moved out into the back yard. We wanted everything to be ready in time, and loved having such a joyful deadline to work towards.

We also began looking further into the future. The baby's due date was one week before Preston's birthday. So we began talking about the 18th and 21st birthdays that would be within one week of each other. I wondered, or rather hoped, that our kids would always be close and excited to celebrate their birthdays together each year.

The excitement was growing and each week was flying by. I felt so blessed and so grateful. I couldn't wipe the smile off my face. I was truly happy and so excited.

# 5

## little mr or little sister?

It was a warm Autumn day and Preston and I were soaking up the sunshine on a picnic blanket in our front garden. He munched down his fruit salad and told me all the things he was going to do with his new baby. From wrestles with daddy and walks on the bike track, to watching Thomas and building lego towers, he had it all planned out.

It made me wonder what his reaction would be if it was a boy or a girl. Was he expecting a little boy to wrestle with, or did he think wrestling his little sister would be just as much fun? For some reason I always thought that we would have at least one boy and one girl, but after having Preston I enjoyed raising a little boy so much that having two boys close together was also a beautiful thought.

In my heart I knew the gender of our baby was decided long ago, and I was so happy with whatever God had planned for our family. That didn't stop me being curious though. I loved thinking about it and trying to guess what our baby would be. We decided to wait until the birth to find out the gender. We loved that anticipation and everyone around us trying to guess.

When I was pregnant with Preston I was surprised by the number of strangers who would tell me what they thought I was having. Some people even referred to the size of my backside as their point of reference. One lady stopped me in the street, spun me around to look at my back and told me it was a boy. Her daughter then told me "she's never wrong you know". She wasn't wrong that time either. But maybe if she chose to look at my stomach to make her presumption, it would have been a little more polite.

I was five weeks pregnant when I called to book an appointment with my midwife. I spoke to her about wanting a natural birth, much different from the emergency c-section I experienced the first time. I was excited to think about what it would be like to have Jonathan there in the room, to share that experience with me. Every time I pictured the birth and the midwife laying my new baby on my chest it was always a boy. Even when I tried to think out a girl scenario in my head, it would always correct itself to be a boy.

I knew I would be happy either way, but in my heart I was pretty certain this was the little brother for my Preston. His very own best buddy to grow and learn and play with. I could already foresee a life of Saturday morning sports. Would it be alongside the soccer field? Would we be rushing off to dancing concerts as well? Or splitting mum and dad between the two? Either way we were pretty sure this baby, boy or girl, would complete our family.

We were looking to the future with so much hope and joy. Despite the complications I had at the end of my pregnancy with Preston it was all smooth sailing up until then. I didn't expect anything would go wrong with this baby. In fact I was more at ease now than ever.

For the first seven weeks of my pregnancy I was blissfully unaware of the nightmare that was to follow. I thought that nothing could take the smile from my face or the joy from my heart.

I was wrong.

# 6

## why are you crying?

There have been very few times in my life that I've literally felt a pain so great in my heart that I knew it was breaking. As I sat in the emergency room alone with tears rolling down my cheeks I felt so incredibly sad, more sad than I had ever been before or ever thought was possible.

Everyone's story is different. There may be some similarities, but each story is unique – just like the cracks in our hearts, just like our babies. The memory of the night we lost our baby is still so strong in my mind, like it only happened yesterday.

It was March 2017. We had a busy weekend with two birthday parties to attend. It was raining all weekend so I was in charge of bringing the 'ball pit' to each party. It had rained for Preston's first birthday so his grandma went out and bought 1700 plastic balls to fill our blow-up swimming pool. It was a big spend for one party, so we often leant them to our friends to borrow for their parties too.

By Sunday morning I was feeling more tired than usual, and my uterus felt really heavy. It felt like I was carrying a bowling ball around under my jeans, and there was a little cramping as well.

16

Something didn't feel right, but I checked it out online and was reassured that these were normal symptoms of early pregnancy.

When I got home from the second party on Sunday night I started bleeding. I rang my midwife and explained the colour and consistency of the blood. At this stage it was quite light in colour and there wasn't much of it. She told me to lay down and rest and keep an eye on it. If the blood became darker or more frequent I should go to the hospital.

Twenty minutes later I was on my way to emergency. The bleeding had continued and I started to panic. I asked Jonathan to stay at home with Preston. It was almost his bed time and I didn't want to leave him with anyone else. I didn't want Preston at home worried about us, or to be up late, waiting around at the hospital.

Even though it meant I would be alone I felt better knowing that he was with his dad. I would have loved Jonathan to be with me, but we still hadn't told our family we were pregnant. I had to be brave. I had to trust God that everything would be ok and go to the hospital alone.

When I got to emergency they let me move ahead of everyone sitting in the waiting room and took me straight inside. I think this gave me a false sense of hope. It made me think that if something was wrong that they could fix it. I was wrong. I sat in that hospital being monitored for four long hours hoping, praying, begging for a miracle.

It was a Sunday night so I was told that the doctors were unable to do a scan to see what was happening. They did a blood test to check my hormone levels. Every time I went to the bathroom I took photos of the blood with my phone so that I could show the doctor when she asked me to describe it.

Whenever I showed her a photo the only thing she would say is "that is a significant amount of blood". I couldn't get anything else out of her. I'm not sure if she was trying to protect me, or if she really didn't know what was happening. Either way there wasn't much compassion. The nurses were busy and I was alone, just waiting.

I messaged my friends Cameron and Tracey from church. I told them I was pregnant and at the hospital, and I asked them to pray for me. Tracey offered to come and sit with me but I told her it was ok. Her prayers were more than enough. It was nice to have this beautiful couple who I could trust, back us in prayer. I was so full of fear, and I knew that I needed them to pray on my behalf. I felt like there was nothing else I could do but wait.

After a couple of hours sitting alone, my mind was a racing mess. I wondered, if I was miscarrying, did this mean that the blood and tissue I could see was the last I would ever see of my baby? My heart literally ached with every flush. I wondered should I be keeping this somehow? If this is my child, shouldn't there be more dignity involved in our baby's last moments than the flush of a public hospital toilet?

After four long hours I had reached my emotional limit. The doctors were doing their shift change-over. I had just experienced a huge bleed in the bathroom. I sat back in my chair, between the old guy struggling to breathe from too many cigarettes, and the young guy with a small piece of glass in his eye, and I burst into tears.

The doctors rushed over but I was crying so much that I couldn't speak. "What's wrong Michelle?" She asked. "Why are you crying?"

I tried to tell her what was wrong but all I could get out in between each sob was "more … bleeding".

That's when they decided to send me home. The doctor said that if I was miscarrying there was nothing they could do. She told me to go home and get some rest, and book in for an ultrasound the next day.

That night in the hospital was hard. Maybe I shouldn't have made the choice to be alone. Maybe it was all too much. There are no words to explain the heartache I felt. The grief was so real. The pain was intense. I didn't feel like the doctors understood my pain at all.

So that made me wonder, would anyone else?

# 7

## trust me

I walked through the dark hospital car park holding in my tears. I didn't want anyone else to see me cry. After the doctor's reaction I didn't have much faith in people to understand how I was feeling. I sat in my car, put my head on the steering wheel and cried the loudest, most gut-wrenching cry I've ever heard myself cry. I couldn't move, I couldn't breathe.

After a few minutes I lifted my eyes and saw a couple heading towards my car. I'm not sure if they had heard me, or if they were just walking past to get to emergency. But I didn't want to talk to them. I wiped my eyes and started my car, still sobbing but desperate to get out of there.

As I drove away my arms and legs became stiff and stopped working properly. My sobbing became uncontrollable again and I began yelling out to God "Please no. Please no." I cried until I couldn't breathe and then cried some more.

When I got home Jonathan met me outside in the driveway. He helped me out of the car and wrapped his arms around me. I just stood there and sobbed into his chest. I don't know how long we were there. It felt like a really long time. No words. Just crying, inconsolable crying.

One of the great things about Jonathan is that he knows when to speak and when to be silent. He is the most honest and genuine person I know (but more on him later). That night on our driveway he didn't try to make everything better. He didn't try to tell me that everything would be ok. He just held on tight. I knew that we were in this together.

We still had no definitive answers. That night was one that I'm sure we will never forget. Trying to stay hopeful while we feared the worst was so difficult. We were both praying for a miracle but with every bleed and cramp it became harder and harder to hold on to that hope.

We went inside and sat on the lounge. I said to Jonathan "God's not talking to me. Usually I can hear Him so clearly, but tonight, He's not saying anything."

That's what scared me the most, and made me expect the worst. All of those hours in the hospital and nothing from God. Was I blocking His voice because I feared bad news? The silence was terrifying.

I decided to take a warm shower. I didn't know if I was brave enough to hear the answer but in between my tears I asked the question anyway: "Lord, where are you? Why aren't you talking to me?"

And then I heard Him say: "Michelle, you're not listening."

Deep down in my heart I knew that I was shutting Him out. I had put up a wall because I was so scared of what He might say and I didn't want to hear it. I think in that situation I wanted to live in false hope that things might be ok, rather than have to face the heart-breaking truth that things weren't.

I closed my eyes. "Ok" I said. "Ok, I'm listening."

Then came the words that reached deep into my soul, "Michelle, I need you to trust me".

In most circumstances this might sound like a good thing, but I knew instantly that it wasn't. I knew in my heart that God didn't mean that I should trust him that my baby was alive and well inside me. He wanted me to trust Him with my heart. I had to trust Him, that after all this was over, His hands would hold every single piece of my heart together for as long as it would take.

He wanted me to trust Him that without my baby, I would be ok. I wasn't sure if I was strong enough for this. I didn't know if I would ever be ok again, but I knew that I had no choice.

This season of my life was such a journey of faith. The purpose of this book was to share my story and give others some hope. I wanted to share with you my experience. This is my own journey of hope and faith, that led me through the darkest time in my life and back out into the light.

If you have recently lost your baby then you might be at the point where you don't want to feel ok yet. It might feel like the pain in your heart is what makes your baby so real. I know that feeling well.

You can't rush grief. But you can have hope. Hope that one day, when you're ready, you will smile and feel normal again. Hope that one day, you will hold your precious babe in your arms. Hope that you will get through this, and that your heart won't always hurt as much as it does right now.

## 8

# broken

I had very little sleep that night. In my heart I knew that my baby was gone. But having no medical proof, I tried hard to hold on to the possibility of a miracle. It was like a bad dream that I couldn't wake up from.

Unable to sleep, I looked online for answers. I began frantically searching for what my HCG (hormone chorionic gonadotropin) level should be and how much it should have risen since my first blood test a few weeks ago.

I was searching things like "how to tell if you are miscarrying", "bleeding and cramping at 7 weeks pregnant", "colour of blood when miscarrying", "how much blood is lost during miscarriage".

I tried to think of everything that I ate in the past week and was even trying to find out if iron tablets could cause a miscarriage because that was the only recent and significant change to my diet.

I felt myself getting desperate. The pain was getting worse with such bad cramping. By the next morning the pain was so intense I could hardly stand up. The physical pain mixed with my emotional anxiety tipped me over the edge. I sat on our dining room floor, doubled over in pain, and burst into tears. I couldn't wait any longer. I asked Jonathan to take me back to the hospital. I needed answers.

At my request, Jonathan dropped me back to emergency and took Preston out for breakfast. I didn't really want to be alone again, but I felt like it was the only way I knew how to be strong, and to protect Preston from the harsh reality of hospitals and sick people.

I called my friend Alicia and she offered to come and stay with me for as long as I needed her. I thanked her but said no. The moment I told her not to come, I realised that a combination of both fear and grief had taken over. My beautiful friend, who had always been there for me, wanted to come and hold my hand, but I turned her away. My fear that she wouldn't understand the depth of what I was feeling, meant that I had to be brave, and was left to go through it alone.

I cried to the triage nurse as I explained what had happened and handed over the doctors report from the night before. She pushed me through to see the doctor pretty quickly. I was there for about an hour before they took more blood to compare with the levels from yesterday. I sat quietly in the emergency recliner, wiping tears from my cheeks with a tissue, and forcing down water to prepare for my scan.

The doctor came in to see me and took me through to the ultrasound room. After a quick ultrasound he said that he couldn't tell what was happening. He said I would need to go to a specialist imaging centre for a proper scan. More false hope. With every unanswered test I tried to hold on to my baby, in hope that things might be ok, but at the same time I knew in my heart it was too late.

I managed to book in a scan for later that afternoon. We went home and played the waiting game. More online searching, more waiting. I kept looking at the photos I took of my blood the night before. Was this really my baby? I knew in my heart that if I had

24

miscarried, my child was already in heaven. But that didn't take the pain away.

My heart was broken. I was broken. I had never felt so unbelievably sad in all my life.

# where's the dignity?

Whilst I struggled with the fact that the physical remains of my baby had been flushed down a public hospital toilet, I was also faced with the reality that some people working in the medical profession struggled with the concept of compassion.

I booked my scan with an imaging centre specialising in 3D images. I hadn't been there before but I was told it would give me a better look into what was happening. I called to book in and explained everything that I had experienced over the past 24 hours. When we arrived, I handed in my referral from the hospital emergency department and waited for my turn.

The waiting room was full of happy pregnant people. Some further along than others. They were chatting away with their husbands, rubbing their bellies, telling their kids to behave in the toy corner. They all had that happy glow, the same glow I had just a few short days ago. They all looked so excited for what they were about to see.

I could tell that for some it was their first scan and some were much further along, almost ready to meet their little bundle of joy.

Watching them was tough. How I longed to swap places. I wanted more than anything for this to be one of those happy routine scans.

I wasn't sure what to expect once I got in the room. I was struggling to process what was happening to us. I sat holding Jonathan's hand until they called my name. As I walked slowly along the creaking wooden floorboards, I could hear Preston's cries as I left him in the waiting room with Jonathan. He wanted to come with me.

With every step I felt my heart climb further into my throat. Was this the moment I would learn the devastating fate of my unborn child? Or would this be the moment that God answered my prayers with a miracle? I had heard stories in the past of people bleeding but their babies were still ok. The answer I'd been waiting on for more than 24 hours was just moments away, and I was terrified.

The nurse started the scan. I stared at the screen intently hoping for a miracle. With every blob on that screen and every measurement she took I wondered if that was my baby. Had all this fear and trauma been for nothing? Would everything be ok after all?

She had a puzzled look on her face. I told her I was so nervous. She ignored me. Then she took out the equipment for an internal ultrasound. Just before she began she asked me: "So you haven't had any pain or bleeding have you?" I couldn't believe what I was hearing.

I told her that the pain and bleeding were the reasons I was there, and explained to her what had happened. To which she replied with an annoyed tone "well this is something you should have told me before we began".

My heart skipped a beat and I held in the tears. I felt like a child who had done something wrong. My voice began to crack as I told her that I explained everything when I booked the appointment, and that it was all written on the referral letter from the hospital. She picked up the letter and said "oh yes I see it on here".

It was very obvious to me that this lady had never lost a child. The experience at this imaging centre only made me more fearful that the rest of the world wasn't going to understand my grief. Her attitude scared me. If someone working in this industry didn't understand how I felt, or know how to show compassion, then how could I expect anyone else to?

I laid there in that dark ultrasound room, sad, angry, annoyed and exhausted. The nurse finished up the scan and turned the screen further towards me so I could see it. "There is nothing there," she said. "Your baby is gone".

*10*

---

# gabriel luca

The weeks that followed shook me to my core. The pain was so intense and I'd never felt grief like this before.

My hormones were a mess. I was constantly crying. It felt like the world I knew would never be the same again. There were days I cried so much that I started to worry if I would ever stop. Was this the new me? Why couldn't I pull it together? Who would want a wife or a mum who was sad all the time, a mum who had lost her joy?

I didn't want to be that person. I didn't want to be the sad girl who cried all the time, but part of me also didn't want to stop crying. Some days it felt like being so sad made my baby more real and kept him in my heart.

I had so much fear that people weren't going to understand my grief. I wanted to tell people what had happened, but at the same time I was terrified of their reaction. If they didn't understand or say the right thing, how would that make me feel?

I was most worried about those closest to me. If the people who loved me most in this world didn't understand my sorrow or give me permission to be sad, then how could I possibly move forward.

A few days after my miscarriage, we went to see Jonathan's parents for my father in-law's 70th birthday dinner. He wasn't having a big party, so this was the only celebration for his birthday. I knew I should be there but at the same time I didn't want to go. I couldn't stop crying and I feared what everyone would say to try and make me feel better. At the same time I was terrified to stay home by myself, I wanted to be close to Jonathan and Preston so I decided to go with them.

When we arrived, Jonathan's dad was cooking outside on the barbecue and his mum was inside in the kitchen. I walked over to his dad and he gave me a hug. Tears welled in my eyes. "You'll be ok," he said and gave me a pat on the back. I smiled and whispered happy birthday as we hugged. So far so good, I had managed to keep it together. We walked inside and Jonathan's mum came over and gave me a strong hug. She held on tight as I burst into tears in her arms. There it was. The grief in my heart had exploded out onto her shoulder, I couldn't hold it in.

We sat down and I told Jonathan's mum what had happened. I told her my baby was flushed down the toilet at the hospital, and my heart went along with him. She took a deep breath. "Your baby went straight to heaven to be with the Lord," she said. "He never made it to the toilet."

She was right, and that was something I needed to remember every time I thought back to that night. My baby died inside me and went straight to heaven. He went from the safe, warm protection of his mother's womb, straight into the arms of Jesus, and I was so grateful for that.

A few days later we decided to tell our friends and family about our baby. We didn't want to go through life pretending he never existed.

To us this baby would always be a part of our family and we wanted to share him with those we loved.

I wasn't sure how our friends would react. I knew that whatever they said, would be said in love, but I really didn't want to hear things like "at least you were only seven weeks pregnant" or "at least it happened naturally and you didn't need a procedure" or "there must have been something wrong with the baby, so this was saving you a lifetime of pain".

I just wanted people to let me be sad, to tell me that it's ok to cry and to give me permission to be sad for as long as I wanted to be. I wanted people to acknowledge my baby, to believe that my sadness was warranted, to understand my heartache was real, and that all my tears were for my lost child.

To help with our grief, Jonathan and I decided that our baby needed a name. We may not have held this sweet child in our arms, but he certainly had a heartbeat, and he was as real to us as Preston was.

I messaged my friend Jenny. It had been three years since she lost her baby boy, Michael, and I knew she would understand my pain. I told her I felt like I had been hit by a bus. We cried back and forth through many messages. She said that naming her son was validation that he did exist, because he did, even if nobody else got to meet him.

After a lot of thought Jonathan and I chose the name Gabriel Luca. The name was so symbolic of what was ahead for us.

Gabriel means God is my strength. I knew that I couldn't go on and be the best mum for Preston, the best wife for Jonathan, the best version of me, without God's strength. Luca means bringer of light. While it was such a dark time for us we still had hope, hope that God would bring light back into our world and heal our hearts.

We sent the name out to our friends and family. I messaged

31

Jonathan's brother Jordan and his girlfriend Katie. Jordan wrote back, "Love it! Gabe the babe!" I read his message and smiled. I pictured Gabriel learning to play soccer with his uncle Jordan, and for a moment, my heart filled with joy.

I wrote Gabriel's name on that first picture Preston drew of our baby and framed it. It sits on the shelf in our bedroom and I look at it every day.

To me it's a beautiful, but sad reminder of our baby and our heartache. It reminds of the hope we had for what could have been, and our hope for all that's still to come.

## 11

## the angel

As each day passed my heart felt heavier, and I started to feel the darkness close in around me. I was caught up in a constant cycle of fear, desperation and hope. I wasn't sure what the future would hold, or if I'd ever be strong enough to risk this happening again. For the first time in my life I felt really broken.

My friend Teresa came to see me. She brought me the most beautiful angel as a gift from my mothers group. She sat on the lounge and I told her about everything that had happened. As I shared my story about the hospital and the name we chose for Gabriel she had tears in her eyes.

She then gave me permission to feel however I needed to feel. She said, "take all the time you need, and if you feel good today but not tomorrow then take some more time. Whatever you feel, even if it changes each minute, it's ok." I was so grateful for this. I felt like taking one minute at a time was all I could do. Looking any further forward was terrifying. There were times when I started to feel strong and thought, "It's ok, I can do this", but then shortly after I would be a blubbering mess again. I was scared to tell people I was doing fine in case the next day or the next hour came and I wasn't fine at all.

We then talked about all the mums in our group who had babies in heaven, and all of their siblings who wouldn't be here today if those babies had made it to this earth. Until now I had never thought of this. My heart was too broken to look into the future and see a precious baby who wouldn't be here if this baby had made it.

After Teresa left, I messaged Julia from our group. She too had experienced a miscarriage before falling pregnant with her daughter Isabel. She told me, that as heartbreaking as it is, she knows that if she hadn't lost her baby, her beautiful little girl wouldn't be here today. Then she said something I'll never forget, "and I can't imagine this world without Isabel in it."

I started to cry. She was right. I couldn't imagine this world without Isabel either, or Thomas, Tyler and Daniel. Four beautiful kids in our mothers group of 12. They had all become Preston's buddies and wouldn't be here today if their amazing mumma's hadn't survived the heartache that I was feeling.

My friend Renee was another brave friend who told me she knew the tremendous pain I was dealing with, but eventually, it made her so grateful for her little boy Emmett, her rainbow baby that came after the dark clouds. My friends were showing me that there was hope, that there could be light after the darkness. It was something I would have to keep in my mind, to help me in the future, but for now I just wanted to be sad for a while. I just needed to feel it.

I had friends dropping in and calling or messaging daily to make sure I was ok. One day, when I was in the pit, my friend Soraiya messaged and told me to "hold on to my faith" to get me through. Her words stuck with me. I was holding on so tight to my faith in

God, and my faith that I would see my child in heaven. No matter how broken I felt, I had to hold on.

I didn't feel angry, just really hurt and sad. I never once questioned God and asked "why me?" I knew this was part of His plan and my baby was safe and loved with Jesus. But still, it hurt so much. I found the nights especially hard. I spent so many hours in bed, crying, weeping for the baby I wanted so desperately to have back inside me. I kept thinking back to that night in the shower and God's words, "Michelle, I need you to trust me."

One night in particular, I felt the grief so heavy in my heart. I couldn't stop crying. I tried to read my bible, I tried to pray. But all I could do was cry out to God, "I trust you Lord but you have to give me something. It hurts so much."

And that's when He said to me:

"Michelle, the angels are singing your baby to sleep".

A flood of tears poured from my face into my pillow, but this time I felt something different.

This one sentence gave me so much peace. Over the years I had heard so many times that the sound of angels singing was the most beautiful sound you could ever imagine. Music had been such a big part of Preston's life. We were always singing him to sleep or playing worship music in the car and at home. I think God knew exactly what to say, that would give me hope and that peace that surpasses all understanding.

I pictured my tiny baby in the arms of an angel being sung to sleep. That's when it hit me. Gabriel was in paradise. He would grow up with Jesus and learn to sing with the angels. He would never have to face the sadness of this world. He would never feel heartache, stress, anxiety or fear. My baby wasn't with me, my heart was broken, but my baby was ok, in fact he was truly blessed.

The next day I received a gift in the mail. My pastor had ordered me a book to read. It was called *Jesse: found in heaven,* and was written by the Pastor of C3 Church Chris Pringle. Chris and her husband Phil lost their first baby through miscarriage.

As I flicked through the pages tears started rolling down my cheeks. Things God had told me the night before were all being confirmed on the pages of this book. She spoke about her baby "cradled in the arms of an angel". She said he was "raised and educated in the courts of heaven.... tutored by angels, saints and, I am sure has walked and talked with Jesus."

I thought back to my prayers the night before and heard it again "Michelle, the angels are singing your baby to sleep."

I didn't know it was possible to feel so sad and yet so grateful at the same time. God was reminding me that my sweet baby was at home, with Him, in heaven.

Sure, my heart was broken, and I knew that every Mother's Day, Christmas and birthdays my heart would feel heavy for the beautiful baby that's not here. But God was holding my heart together. I am full of so much hope and I am so grateful, that because of my faith I will get to see my baby again. He will have grown up in heaven, but Gabriel will still know who his mum and dad are. He will know how much we love him and our sweet child will be the second person waiting in line to see us when we get there.

What a beautiful day that will be.

In her book Chris Pringle also encouraged her readers to write about their own experiences as part of the healing process. I had already started writing our story in my journal and this encouraged me to keep going.

A few days later, Preston and I went to visit some local nuns to take them some groceries. We took a walk around their prayer garden and

I found a sign that said "Lord, I don't understand you, but I trust you." It made my heart skip a beat. I whispered that line into the breeze and felt that peace covering me again. Not only was I trusting God to take care of my child, I was trusting Him that I would be ok and I was trusting in the big picture.

Jonathan's beautiful nan in Mount Gambier sent me a card after we lost our baby. She wrote … "I am so sorry to hear of your loss. I do hope God has helped you to deal with this loss and helped with the healing. We don't have all the answers why certain things happen, but God sees the big picture and we don't, we just see a small part."

She put it so simply, but it's so true. We don't see the big picture, but we can have hope in the big picture. God knew what I needed to hear when I was at my lowest. I literally cried out to Him and with a few words He filled me with so much hope and peace. Death had lost its sting, and it didn't stop there.

A few weeks later I ran into my beautiful friend Lauren. I told her about Gabriel and she asked me if I had given myself time to grieve properly. I told her what the Lord said about the angels singing my baby to sleep. She gave me the biggest hug and said "Have you heard angels singing? I'll send you the link."

A singer in America, named Jason Upton, was recording a song called "Fly" when a second voice began singing behind him. I searched online for the song when I got home and one of the band members shared their experience. When I heard the angels voice I became so overwhelmed. God used my gorgeous friend and that song to remind me of how real He is, and to give me that big picture perspective. I might not understand why I had to lose my baby, but I do have peace in my heart. It might take time, but I know that Gabriel is ok and I have faith that one day I will be too.

# 12

## jonathan

It's safe to say that the greatest blessing in my life has always been Jonathan. After losing Gabriel, I felt a much deeper love for my husband, and I was even more grateful for him than ever before. I'm not sure what I would have done without his love and support through this journey. I dedicated this book to him, because without him I wouldn't be the person I am today and this book would never have been written.

I met Jonathan in 2006. We were both working at the local newspaper. He was the photographer and I was the journalist. I loved working with him. It was always such an adventure, out on the road, looking for the best story, chasing the news as it broke.

I was absolutely smitten from the moment we met. Jonathan on the other hand was a little more reserved. He wasn't keen on dating a girl he worked with, just in case things didn't work out. Even after we decided to take the plunge and become a couple there was no kissing, holding hands or flirting during work hours. He always kept his cool, like a seasoned professional.

As a human being I'd say that Jonathan is one of the best. He has a beautiful soul. He is quiet when he needs to be, but will speak out against anything that isn't right. He is one of those guys who doesn't talk just for the sake of it, so when he is speaking you know it's worth listening to. He's sensitive and compassionate. He's talented, artistic and has a great eye for detail.

He works hard and is always so dedicated to doing the best he can, whether it's at work, renovating our house or being the best husband and dad he can be. I'm not sure what I would do without him. He is my rock, my moral compass, my true love, my soul mate.

No matter how good or bad things get, I always take time to thank God that He blessed me with Jonathan. Since I was a little girl all I ever wanted was to grow up and marry someone as awesome as him. I love living this life together and I am so grateful for him every single day.

When we lost Gabriel, Jonathan stepped up to the plate. He took time off work and supported me physically and emotionally. I was in so much pain that I could barely move off the lounge. He kept the house running: cooking, cleaning and chasing after Preston.

He protected me from people who might possibly do or say something to upset me. He supported all the things I wanted to do to remember our baby. He showed his love every minute of every day, even when words were hard to find.

I worried about him too. I wasn't sure how sad he was feeling or if he needed to talk about it. I hoped that all my tears wouldn't stop him from being able to open up and tell me how he felt. There were times when Jonathan would tell me that he didn't know what to say to make things better. I remember pushing my forehead into his chest, my tears soaking his shirt and saying, "just pray babe," and that's what he did.

He hadn't connected with our baby like I had, but he did say that it was hard to see me so sad when we lost Gabriel. I know that he was praying for me, and that those prayers got me through that devastating time.

Through all the tears and heartache I just kept thinking "Thank God for Jonathan" or "Thank God he's not at work this week". I really needed him there to help me. No matter what happens in my life I am just so grateful that we have each other, and that all of my children get to have him as their dad. He's the best.

## 13

## will it hurt like this forever?

We sat at the table quietly eating dinner. Jonathan was sitting across from me and Preston was between us at the head of the table. I pushed the carrots around my plate for a while, then out of nowhere I burst into tears.

I couldn't hold it in. The pain was too much.

Jonathan looked at me and reached across the table to hold my hand. I looked up at him and whispered "Will it hurt like this forever?" Jonathan opened his mouth to speak, but before he could answer Preston looked at Jonathan's hand, grabbed my other hand and said "No mummy. Nothing hurts forever."

I smiled at him and cried some more. I didn't know if he was right. I wanted to believe that that one day I'd be able to get through my dinner without crying, and that it wouldn't always hurt this much.

The pain I felt in my heart seemed to be amplified by the fear I had that others wouldn't know why I was so sad. I was terrified that people wouldn't understand my grief. How could I expect them to understand? They had never met my baby or felt the same love inside like I had.

41

Maybe if our baby had lived even a short while, and our friends and family got to meet him or hold him in their arms, then they might feel the same grief that we do. After all, nobody even knew I was pregnant. How could I expect them to feel the same pain I was feeling? How could I expect them to understand or react to my pain the way I needed them to.

I walked into church on Sunday morning to a sea of smiling faces. My brain was in a fog and I wasn't sure who knew that we had lost our baby. As I held back the tears and looked for a seat, I tried to avoid eye contact and small talk with everyone. I wasn't sure how I would react if somebody asked me if I was ok. As the worship music started playing I suddenly felt my friend Janelle wrap her arms around me so tight. Her long curly hair hid my face as I cried into her shoulder.

I remembered her telling me years ago how she felt when she lost her baby through miscarriage. I could feel her hug was a hug that knew my pain. She didn't say anything, just kept squeezing tighter. When the embrace finally ended she wiped the tears from my face and hugged me again. I didn't need her to say anything. I knew that she had felt the darkness I was feeling for herself. I also knew that with the help of the Lord she had come through the valley and ended up with two beautiful children of her own.

In that moment I wondered how she did it. The pain in my heart was still so intense, and I found it hard to look forward to a time when I would be able to smile or laugh like I used to, let alone try for another baby. Part of me wanted to fast-forward to a time when the grief was less overwhelming, so I could breathe again. The other part of me wanted to lock myself in my room and be sad forever.

My beautiful sister-in-law Peta sent me a link to an article about miscarriage the next day. It basically gave me permission to be sad, and it validated how I was feeling. I remember it said that my grief was warranted and my baby was real and it was ok to cry and feel sad for as long as I needed to. As I read it I felt this release and I realised there were so many other mums out there feeling how I was.

As part of my healing process I decided to book in some counselling. I had some prayer sessions with the leaders at my church and also went to see my psychologist. The first session was only a few days after my miscarriage. I didn't get many words out to begin with. I mostly just cried. My counsellor's name was Alyson and she is such a beautiful human being. She is a Christian lady who was so compassionate and supportive. There's been a few times now that I've shared my heart about Gabriel only to see a tear in her eye.

She's someone I can be honest with, without feeling any judgement. I've had so much fear about Preston suffering with the same anxiety issues that I did growing up and she has helped me through that. It's not good to live in fear. It can be so debilitating. I didn't want this experience to be one that brought more fear into our lives, especially when it came to our future pregnancies and children.

Talking to Alyson about our baby was really helpful. She told me that the pain I felt might always be there, but it wouldn't always be as intense as it was now. This helped me a lot. She also validated the pain that I was feeling. She knew how real my baby was and that the feelings I had were warranted because I had just lost a child.

She also told me it that was ok to do things that would keep Gabriel's memory alive which was something I worried about. I told her I didn't want to ever forget him. I was even scared to fall pregnant again in case that felt like I was replacing Gabriel. Aside from the picture Preston drew, I wrote down a few things that I wanted to do to remember our baby.

When I'm ready, I want to buy a Christmas bauble with Gabriel's name on it for our Christmas Tree. Preston can help me hang it up every year. I also think Gabriel's due date will be when we celebrate his birthday. I think it would be nice to bake a cake together. I didn't want to put too much pressure on myself though. I decided to make these plans but I would wait to see how I felt. I can only imagine this first year that the due date would be a tough one to get through.

The following morning, after I cried into my plate at the dinner table, I took Preston to his swimming lesson. In hindsight this wasn't the best idea. I thought maybe doing something normal would help me. It was so surreal to sit on the side of the pool, in the same seat I sat in a week before when I was pregnant and happy. This week I was cramping, bleeding and broken. Yet I still smiled at Preston every time he looked at me for assurance that he was doing a good job.

About half way through the lesson Preston started crying. He was inconsolable, calling out "mummy" and went from quietly waiting for his turn on the edge of the pool to hanging from his teacher's neck sobbing into her shoulder. It started to become clear to me that I wasn't the only one suffering. Preston could sense something was wrong. Normality seemed so far away for all of us. As I pulled out of the car park, Preston sobbing in the back seat, I decided that once we got home I was never leaving the house ever again.

## 14

## the stutter

As a mum, my heart was aching for the beautiful baby we lost, and all the things that could have been. It was also aching for Preston. Through all of this I was so worried about him seeing me so sad all the time. I was concerned about what impact this would have on him. There were so many elements to my grief.

The first two weeks I cried so much. I was still in a lot of pain and my heart ached like never before. I spent a lot of time on the lounge in tears. No matter how hard I tried not to get upset in front of Preston he saw me cry a lot.

He's such a beautiful little boy. So loving and sensitive. Even some cartoons would have him in tears. I remember in the past we had to turn off an episode of Thomas the Tank Engine because he got so upset when Thomas derailed and spilt his load of cheese all over the tracks. I was conscious of what effect seeing me this way could have on his little heart.

Whenever I cried, Preston would come over and pat my back or give me a hug. "Mummy a bit sick" he would say. I know he was only two, but he could tell that something was wrong. He used to always talk about the baby in my belly, but suddenly that stopped as well.

Then during the times I was feeling ok, and the tears had stopped, he would run over with a big smile and ask "mummy all better?". It must have been so confusing for him. I could see he was struggling with it. He was a little more quiet than usual and a bit more clingy to his dad.

Then one morning he woke up with a stutter. It usually happened when he was saying mummy. If it was at the start of the sentence we would get "mu mu mum mu mum mummy". Every time it happened my heart ached for him and I blamed myself for letting him see me so sad.

What had I done? I had read it's ok to be sad in front of your kids so they could learn about emotions, and know that it's ok to cry when you're sad. But had I let it go too far or for too long? Had my sadness caused this?

The stutter went on for a couple of days and it got worse and worse. His speech started to get stuck on more and more words. My heart was broken. I didn't want him to suffer. He was obviously struggling with the grief and seeing me so upset.

We took Preston to the community nurse for an assessment. We told her everything that had happened. She looked at me and said "Michelle this is not your fault". I burst into tears. I didn't believe her of course, but it was nice of her to say. She said that Preston was very bright and aside from the stutter his speech and vocabulary were quite advanced for his age. She said she thought the stutter would stop eventually on its own, but she could get the speech pathologist to call me if I was worried.

When I spoke to the speech pathologist she told me that sometimes stutters can start after an emotional or traumatic time but sometimes kids just wake up one day and start stuttering. She also said it could stop on its own, but if Preston got stuck on words and couldn't move on and began getting very emotional or upset about it we should call back.

I really can't put in to words how worried I was. My emotions were already in overdrive. We had been through so much and I hated that this could be the cause for his stutter.

I was so upset. That's when I made the decision to cut back the days at my new job. If this whole experience taught me anything it was how important my family was to me. My boss was so lovely and gave me a lap top to work from home. I spent more time at home and tried my best to get myself and Preston back into a routine. My tears became less frequent and it began to feel like things were getting a little closer to normal again.

I wanted to share this chapter because there's a chance you might be going through something similar. Maybe not a stutter, maybe you're just worried about being sad all the time in front of your kids. I felt so guilty for what Preston was going through, but eventually everything did turn out ok. In hindsight, Preston saw his mum with a broken heart and then he saw his mum get better and stronger each day.

There have been a few days with more tears than others but he saw me get through those days as well. He knows how strong his mum is, and that it's ok to cry, it's ok to be sad and it doesn't mean you'll be sad forever.

# 15

## p is for preston

I sat on the lounge under a blanket for days, I felt stuck, unable to move, and like a dark cloud was hovering over me. I had cancelled all of our plans so I wouldn't need to leave the house. I felt particularly sad about missing dinner with my high school girlfriends. My beautiful friend Jess was visiting from Adelaide and I was desperate to see her and all the girls. But there was no way I could face a restaurant full of people, or any kind of socialising. I told Jess I was sorry, but I felt so broken and sad and I just needed to be alone and sleep.

That afternoon Preston was in the toy room playing with Jonathan when I heard a knock at my door. I slowly walked through the entrance way, expecting to see the postman, but to my surprise it was Jess standing there with a bunch of native flowers from her mums garden. I opened the door and burst into tears. She hugged me tight. "I know you don't want any visitors so I won't stay long," she said. "I just had to see you."

I made her come in and sit down. Even though I had cancelled on her, I was so happy she ignored me and came anyway. I could see in her eyes that her heart was aching for me. She had to see me for herself. She had to make sure that I knew how much she loved me and cared about me. In that moment I knew that I would do the same for her.

Sometimes when we are struggling with our own grief, it's hard to even think about what others might be feeling as well. My brother and his girlfriend Jess offered to come and visit to help out with Preston. I told them they didn't need to come, but they said they wanted to come to make sure I was ok. I'm glad they came. I'm not sure what it is, but I always feel more peace in my heart when my brother is in the room, and his girlfriend has such a beautiful heart, just like he does. Even though I kept most people away, I found it good to let those closest to me come along beside us, to show their love.

My mum came down to stay with us shortly after we lost Gabriel. She arrived on Saturday, and spent the day playing with Preston while I rested. After Preston went to bed, mum joined us on the lounge with her tissues in one hand and a gift box in the other. I was nervous about what it might be. She was always a thoughtful gift-giver, and I was worried that in my current state my reaction might not be up to scratch.

When I opened the box I saw a beautiful bracelet and some charms inside including the letters G and P. When she gave me the box she began explaining that she added the P for Preston and she started to cry. That's when I realised that her heart was broken too. Not just broken for me, and the pain I was feeling, but also broken for the little baby that she would never get to hold, or shower with love, like she did Preston. She loved him so much and their bond has always been a special one.

I loved the bracelet and the charms, because it was another acknowledgement that my baby was as real to somebody else as he was to me. It meant so much to me that Gabriel's name wasn't only written in heaven, and in my heart, but in somebody else's heart as well. I still haven't been brave enough to get the charms out of the box. Every time I try, I end up standing in my wardrobe crying. I'm glad I have them in there though, waiting for me. They remind me how much my babies are loved by their grandma, and how much I am loved too.

Our friends and family were such a beautiful support during this time. After we said goodbye to Gabriel our house was full of flowers and gifts. Our fridge was full of home-made meals and vegetable-box deliveries. My friend Hayley brought me a guardian angel pin which I treasured. I felt it was a reminder from heaven, that angels were singing my baby to sleep. One day I opened my front door to find a small gift bag sitting on my welcome mat. It was from my friend Alecia. I opened the box to find the most beautiful necklace with a large circle and small circle joined together. It made me burst into tears. She said it represented a mum, always being connected to her baby. It was another validation that my tears were for a baby that may not be here in my arms, but would always be in my heart.

A few days later the postman dropped off another special gift from my friend Renee. It was a plush puppy dog for Preston. As soon as we opened the parcel it was in his arms and never left his sight. "Woofy" as Preston affectionately called him, was a beautiful distraction for our little boy. He took him everywhere he went and to bed each night. Woofy has remained his favourite ever since, especially at bed time.

I know that it's not always the case that people are so understanding and supportive. I wanted to share this chapter because our friends' reactions really helped with our grief. I know not everybody understands the heartache. To be honest, I didn't understand the pain until I felt it myself. We were very blessed to have so many people acknowledge our pain. They might not have understood what we were feeling, or felt like they knew exactly what to do, or say, but they all tried. They all showed love in some way or another. We felt so loved and that made us feel like our baby was loved by them too, and to us that meant the world.

## 16

# the fat controller

There's a photo of our family that is bittersweet for me. It was taken one week after we lost Gabriel. The photo is of Jonathan, Preston and I standing in front of Thomas the Tank Engine with the Fat Controller.

We had purchased tickets for the Thomas Big Day Out with Jonathan's family months in advance. Preston loved Thomas and was so excited to go for a ride on a steam train and meet all of his favourite characters, including the Fat Controller.

My cramping had stopped before the event but I still wasn't sure if my heart could take it. I knew that I would have to hold my tears in for the day, maybe that would be good for me.

I still worried that people didn't understand my grief. I thought that if I made it through the day without crying, everyone would think that I was ok, when really I wasn't. I remember wondering if our family would think that I wasn't sad anymore? Was it too soon to do something so normal? Was Gabriel watching me from heaven thinking that I was strong and courageous, or would he think his mum had forgotten him already?

My mind was a mess and my heart was heavy. I decided to go along to the Thomas Day for Preston. He had been looking forward to it for so long. I didn't want him to miss out and I also didn't want to miss out on seeing him so excited and happy. Sometimes you just have to be strong. There were days when I couldn't leave the house. But this was a day I made myself do it. I cried underneath my sunglasses most of the way there and all the way home. But I managed to hold it together while we were there.

Preston loved riding on Toby. He got to sit in the front seat with his cousin Elijah and watch the driver do his thing. A couple of times I took him for a walk away from the group and the two of us took a ride by ourselves. It was nice. I remember looking at him and feeling so grateful that he was ok. I thought about his birth and how we nearly lost him too. But he was always meant to be here. As Toby chugged along, back and forth between the stations, Preston all of a sudden started yelling "Fat Controller! Fat Controller!" pointing out the window at the long line of people waiting to have their photo taken with him in front of Thomas. Jonathan met us at the station and we joined the queue.

As we lined up I realised that I would somehow have to smile for this photo. I would have to do it for Preston, because one day I would be ok again, and this photo would remind me of how strong I can be, despite how broken I felt at the time. We got to the front of the line and Jonathan's mum took my camera to take the photo. Preston was excited but a little shy to be so close to one of his favourite characters. We said hello to the Fat Controller and smiled for our photo. It's the first time in my life that I felt myself smiling on the outside and crying on the inside.

I know that this photo of our family will always bring some heartache when I look at it. But I'm glad we did it. I think it shows just how strong a mum can be. My heart was smashed into a million pieces that day and I was still bleeding. But that photo shows a family (and the fat controller) standing together with big smiles and a shy but excited two-year-old boy.

It goes to show that we don't always know what people are going through, or what people are hiding beneath their smiles. Standing on that platform I wondered how long I would feel this way. How much longer would I have to be strong? When would I actually feel ok? Or would I just have to start faking it?

## 17

---

## faking it

Ultrasounds when you're pregnant are usually so exciting. I remember the joy I would feel each time I got to see Preston moving around on the screen. Much like how the sound of his heartbeat made me feel whenever I visited my midwife.

A few days after the bleeding stopped my doctor sent me for another ultrasound to make sure my miscarriage had completely occurred naturally. A friend of mine gave me some good advice, and told me to view this scan as purely medical. I had been through so much already that attaching any emotion to this ultrasound would only cause more pain. She was right.

For this scan I had to forget all past experiences, both good and bad. I went to a different scanning centre from the last one, and took my seat in the waiting room. An older lady was there waiting for her scan. She was knitting a blue cardigan for a baby and told me she had a new grandson on the way. She started chatting about her health issues. I can't remember what was wrong with her, but to be honest I didn't mind the distraction at the time. I listened to her talk about the pain she was in, then she moved on to talk about all of her children and grandchildren.

Unfortunately she soon ran out of things to talk about and the subject turned to me. She asked if I was pregnant. I couldn't think quick enough to make up another illness that would require an ultrasound, so I faked a smile and said yes. I didn't have the strength to tell her my story. We had just met and I would probably never see her again. I forced a smile to look happy and excited and hoped the conversation was over.

Then she asked how far along I was. "Seven weeks" I said and faked another smile. What a fraud. I wandered if the cracks were showing. I wondered if she could see right through me. Don't cry, don't cry, hold it together, I kept thinking to myself.

Faking it is hard, but I felt it would be much easier than the alternative. Part of me wanted to let it all out, to tell this stranger that my beautiful baby wasn't here anymore, to let her know that this scan would break my heart all over again because the screen would be empty. I wanted her to know that I never got a photo of this baby to keep, because we lost him too soon, and that this scan was just another confirmation that my hopes and dreams of growing our family had been smashed and put on hold.

I really wasn't looking forward to this scan, but at the same time I wanted to get in there and get it done. Not just to get away from the lady in the waiting room, but so I could start moving forward. I had no idea what that would feel like or what the future held for us, but I knew it would have to happen.

A happy pregnant couple then emerged from the ultrasound room with grandma beside them. They were laughing and the mum had a huge smile on her face. They said they were in shock because their scan a few months ago showed that they were having a baby girl, but this scan confirmed it was actually a boy. The mum said that she thought it was a boy all along, and that's why she hadn't bought any clothes yet. The grandma on the other hand said she had a few pretty dresses to return.

The knitting lady chimed in and asked a million questions. She went through all of her pregnancies and explained that she wasn't very good at guessing the genders of her babies. Then she told them I was seven weeks pregnant and kindly pointed out that it was too early for me to find out if I was having a boy or a girl. They asked if I was going to find out the gender. I said no.

It did make me wonder if my mum intuition was on point? Was I like the mum who knew it was a boy all along only to have it confirmed? Or was I like the knitting lady with no clue? Would I get to heaven and find a beautiful young lady there to greet me, or would Gabriel be the handsome young man I pictured him to be? Only time would tell.

As they called me in for my ultrasound the knitting lady called out "good luck". I know she meant with my pregnancy, but the sentiment rang true. I didn't really need luck though, it was more a case of courage for this one.

I laid on that table praying that she would be gone when I got out. I had done all the faking I could for today and knew that if she asked me how the scan went I would burst into tears. The nurse began the scan and I took a deep breath and looked up at the screen. It was blank. I started crying. "I'm sorry," I said. She took my hand and held it tight.

By this stage a blank screen was considered a blessing because it meant I didn't need a medical procedure to complete the miscarriage, but it still hurt. This ultrasound made it final; that blank screen was my sign to move forward. But did I even want to move forward?

I told the nurse how I had I faked it in the waiting room. After my scan she left the room before I did. I'm not sure if she went out and had the knitting lady moved to a different waiting area, but she was gone when I came out. I was relieved.

Faking it to a stranger before my scan was easy, but months later it felt much harder to do. There are some friends we didn't tell about Gabriel and when they ask when Preston is going to get a brother or sister I feel like I have to fake it all over again.

Sometimes it tears me up inside and I tell them about Gabriel. Other times I stay silent because it hurts way too much, or because I know their reaction will either be awkward or over the top. There were times it was easier to tell the truth, but most of the time I found faking it was best for my broken heart.

# 18

there's no clocks in heaven

Throughout those first few weeks we had regular catch ups with our pastor from Lifehouse Church. Pastor Paul Stevens had become a very close friend of our family over the years and a great support to both Jonathan and myself.

Paul is a former professional football player, he loves people and always has a massive smile on his face. He is a kind man, so compassionate and always speaking life and hope into those around him.

Pastor Paul married us in 2012 and has always been there for our family. When we met up after I lost the baby, I asked Paul if he could pray for my broken heart and against any fear for future pregnancies.

I also shared that I felt like Gabriel was a boy and this made me feel like a boy was missing from our family. I felt like I started to desire another boy, a little brother for Preston and I worried that this desire could grow so strong in my heart that I would only want a boy. What if my next baby was a girl?

Paul gave some great advice. He said I should try not to think of Gabriel as "missing" from our family. "He's very much a part of your family," Paul said. "He's just in heaven, in paradise, like he's on an extended holiday."

Then he said something that I still think back to all the time, "You can ask Jesus to tell your baby you love him any time you want, and He will do that."

Wow. A direct line to my baby. All I had to do was pray. I could ask Jesus to hold Gabriel and tell him that his mummy loves him so much. I loved this idea.

Paul continued to share with us and what he said next gave me so much comfort. "There's no clocks in heaven Mish," he said. "Time doesn't exist. You might be down here waiting 60 years to see Gabriel but when you get there, he's going to feel like he just got there yesterday. There's no concept of time, no fear, no sadness. You're waiting for your baby, but he isn't waiting for you. He knows you, he loves you and knows how much you love him, but he doesn't have the same concept of time or waiting that we do."

No clocks in heaven. The concept blew my mind. We speak of eternity so often and it can be quite difficult to wrap our heads around what it's going to be like. To learn there is no concept of time really took a weight off my shoulders.

I love that my baby isn't sad or missing me like I miss him. I love that he doesn't spend every day wishing his mum would hurry up and get there. I am glad that he doesn't ache to have his mum hold him in her arms the same way my heart aches to hold him.

My eternal perspective is something that has strengthened since losing our child. I've always believed in heaven, but to think of my child growing up in heaven has certainly deepened this perspective. I've researched different people's experiences of heaven and there are some amazing stories from people around the world.

One in particular was the story of Colton Burpo who visited

heaven during an emergency surgery when he was four years old. Over the following months he told his parents stories that he could never have known without having this experience. He even told them about meeting his sister in heaven, a little girl who was a miscarried baby that his parents had never told him about.

The book is called *Heaven is For Real* and I recommend it to anyone who is looking for that hope and peace following the loss of a child.

During his trip to heaven Colton says that he sat on Jesus' lap. His dad then spent months showing Colton hundreds of pictures of Jesus to see what he looked like. Colton would reply with things like, no that's not right, his eyes are the wrong colour or his hair's not right.

One day Colton and his dad saw a news broadcast featuring 8-year-old Akiane Kramarik. She was talking about painting her visions of heaven, including images of Jesus. Colton saw her paintings and said "that's him dad, that's Jesus". Hearing these perceptions of heaven from two children who have never met each other was so interesting to me and I've never forgotten it.

Also in the book Colton tells his parents that there are no old people in heaven, there are only children and young adults. He even points out a photograph of his grandfather aged around 30 and says he saw his poppy in heaven. This made me think, would our baby grow up in heaven, so that by the time we see him he would be in his 20s or 30s? I now had a wonderful image to hold on to, of me getting to heaven to receive a hug from my child, who had grown up in paradise.

I read the book *Heaven is for Real* and I saw the movie before Preston was born. When we lost Gabriel I immediately thought back to Colton Burpo meeting his sister in heaven. God had planted that image in my heart long before I would need it. I'm so glad He did.

In developing our eternal perspective we can strengthen our hearts. We can take our place as children of God long before we get to heaven. We can rest in the knowledge that our time on earth is so short. Sure, I will be apart from Gabriel for the next 60 years or so, but then I get to spend an eternity with him and all the people I love.

If you are new to Christianity or don't know much about it, I encourage you to look further into this eternal perspective and heaven.

Heaven connects us to our beautiful babies, it will allow us to see them again.

# 19

## baby joseph

Jonathan's sister Peta and her husband Rob were almost nine months pregnant when we lost Gabriel. I hadn't told Peta that we were pregnant yet. The plan was to wait until we were about eight weeks and then share the news with them. I love Peta so much and I was so excited that our babies would be so close in age.

There was only seven months difference between Preston and his cousin Elijah. So the thought of our next two babies being seven months apart as well was so special. Preston and Elijah love each other so much. They are best friends and love playing together.

When I saw Peta for the first time after losing our baby I can't say there wasn't a sting. I looked at her belly with different eyes from before. Not eyes of anger or resentment, it just made me feel sad. Sad that my baby wasn't on his way to be friends with her baby. Sad that the gap would now be much bigger between her baby and my next one.

I also felt sad that my aunty experience could be a little different this time. I wondered if I would ever be able to hold her baby without that sting in my heart. Would I be able to show this baby as much love as I did to Elijah? Would this child be the one who always reminded me how old Gabriel would be if he was still here with us, and would that be a good thing or a bad thing?

Spending time with Peta while she was pregnant wasn't as difficult as I thought it might be, it was just different. As it got closer to her due date I began to wonder how I would handle seeing her at the hospital. I really wanted to be ok with it. I wanted to be able to show her and her baby all the love I could. I desperately didn't want things to be different, but I also knew that I shouldn't be too hard on myself and I should allow myself to feel whatever I was feeling.

We got the call that her baby was born and my heart filled with all sorts of emotions. God had started giving me some peace about my baby, so I was in a better place to manage any pain if it came. When I arrived at the hospital my mind began to race. Jonathan was at work so Preston and I headed into the maternity ward alone. I wondered how I would feel when I saw the baby. Would I be ok? Would all those feelings come back? Would I burst into tears? Then what about Preston? How would I explain this to him? I took a deep breath and hoped that I was brave enough to get through the visit.

We walked into Peta's room and all my fears disappeared as I saw the most beautiful little boy in her arms. My heart was so full of love and I felt so much joy for my beautiful sister and her family. They called him Joseph. He was very cute and I instantly fell in love with him. Peta asked me how I was feeling. She was so understanding and compassionate for what I had been through. She told me that it was ok for me not to stay long if it was too hard for me, and that whatever I needed to do would be ok.

I think the hardest thing for me was seeing Preston with Joseph. He was so excited and loved him so much. He wanted to hold the baby so we let him have a cuddle. Preston was so gentle and kept kissing Joseph on the head. Every now and then he would look up at us and say "he's so cute" with a big grin on his face.

It was great to see him so good with babies, but it did bring some heartache. The gap between Preston and his brother or sister was growing. I wondered if he would still love our next baby as much if he was a bit older? How long should we wait before trying again? Baby Joseph was a beautiful reminder of what joy a new baby would bring, not only for me and Jonathan but for Preston as well. He was also a reminder that this joy had been put on hold for us, for a while, and that was ok. I guess it had to be.

I am pleased to say that from the moment we met, I found it very easy to love little Joey despite what I had been through. I love our cuddles and while he reminds me of what could have been it doesn't take away from the aunty love in my heart.

It turns out baby Joseph was a blessing in so many ways and the conversation starter for Preston to ask me about our baby. Not long after he was born I was putting Preston to bed one night. We were talking about how aunty Peta used to have baby Joseph in her belly. That's when he said "Where's mummy's baby gone?" My heart hit my throat. I knew I wanted to have this conversation with him at some point, I just didn't realise it would be so soon.

I sat with him and told him that mummy's baby had gone to heaven to be with Jesus. Preston was well aware of Jesus. Whenever anyone asked him "Where's Jesus?" Preston would answer "in my heart" and touch his chest with both hands. So when I told him our baby went to heaven to be with Jesus, he touched his chest, smiled and said "Jesus in my heart, mummy's baby in my heart."

My heart stopped for a moment and my eyes filled with tears. I smiled and said "That's right beautiful boy. Jesus and mummy's baby will always be in your heart."

## 20

# period

The first period back after my miscarriage was a nightmare. I wasn't actively thinking of Gabriel, or that this period shouldn't be happening, but the hormones and probably the subconscious thoughts had me spiralling down into a pit of darkness.

For the week leading up to my period I was a mess. The crying started again and didn't stop. I could feel my heart was in pieces. I felt so broken, almost like it was happening all over again. Of course when it rains it pours. That week also threw at me some other problems. Some comments made by friends of mine hit a nerve and pressed on some fears that I had been carrying for a long time.

I felt like I was being tested. So many of my relationships were struggling. I couldn't tell if I was over-reacting to a situation because of what I had been through, or if things were actually just getting worse and worse. I felt alone and in darkness. I cancelled all the plans we had that week. I felt so sad and just didn't feel like being around other people again.

My uni friends and their families were supposed to come to our house for dinner. It had been so long since we had seen each other and everyone was looking forward to it. But as the time got closer I began to dread it. Preston was still stuttering and I didn't want him to be surrounded by a big group of people and feel overwhelmed. I didn't want anyone to ask me about his stuttering either.

Don't get me wrong. My uni friends are amazing and supportive, and they have always been there for me. But I could tell I was super sensitive and was getting upset over the simplest things. I just needed some time alone. I didn't want to risk it. I didn't want to put our friendship in jeopardy. I love them too much for that. I told them I wasn't well and cancelled. A good decision, but one I wished I didn't have to make.

This was a really dark time for me. I cried myself to sleep most nights. I remember Jonathan asking me what was wrong, which made me even sadder. Did he think I had forgotten and was ok already? It had only been four weeks. Looking back now I don't think he had forgotten at all. It's totally ok to ask someone what's wrong when they cry, but my mind was a mess, my heart was broken.

My friend Tuyet messaged to see if I was ok. She asked if she could come and see me but I said no. She could tell I wasn't coping. Tuyet sent me the most beautiful prayer asking the Lord to sustain me with an extra portion of strength because my strength was faltering. When I read her message the words extra portion stood out to me. So often we pray for an extra portion with things like our finances or our hearts desires, but Tuyet was right. She could see I needed an extra portion of strength just to survive.

I wanted to include this chapter because I was surprised how much this week and this period affected me. Before this time I was starting to feel like I could function again. Like I was moving forward and looking to the future. But this week really shocked me. I felt like I was experiencing that initial grief and sadness all over again.

It won't be like this for everyone. But if it is, please know that you won't always feel this darkness surrounding you. There are ways out of it. It's good to talk to someone and try not to be too hard on yourself. If you need to cancel plans or spend some time alone, then do what you have to do. Your grief will come and go. I wish I was more prepared for that.

I found being at home with my boys the most peaceful option for me. Preston was such a little ray of sunshine. There were so many times throughout the day that he would say or do something that would make us laugh. Every morning when he woke up he would climb out of his bed and open his curtains. Then from our room we would hear him yell out, "It's morning time!" He would race in and say, "It's ok to get up now guys because it's morning!"

One day I woke up and felt like I was in total darkness, I was in so much pain and just wanted to cry from the minute my eyes opened. I wished it was all a bad dream. Then I heard his little voice call out "It's morning time!" so excitedly.

My little Preston was so excited for a new day. I longed for the day that I would feel like that again. I couldn't imagine how a new day would excite me and make me want to jump out of bed. I gave myself permission to stay in bed that day, but I knew in my heart that through Preston, God was reminding me that one day I would wake up full of joy again. Just not today.

# *21*

---

# breathe

As much as I wanted to allow myself time to grieve, I soon reached the point where I was tired of feeling so sad, and just wanted to breathe again. It was Friday morning and with the weekend approaching I felt like I needed to get out of the house.

Our local showground would be a buzz on Saturday with the annual country show. There would be rides, animals, stalls, show bags and plenty to take my mind off things.

I messaged my friend Leah, a true country girl at heart. We were best friends in Kindergarten and she has been riding horses and living the country life since she could walk. Leah didn't have any children, making her a super fun and adoring aunty to Preston. She loved playing with him and I knew she would have the energy to help me chase him around the show.

I hadn't had the chance to tell her about Gabriel yet. It was something I wanted to tell her face to face. Even though she wasn't a church-goer Leah and I often had long conversations about my faith. I loved sharing stories with her about how God has changed my life or the work He was doing in me. We often swapped books and shared our hearts on the spiritual element of my faith.

I decided I would tell her about Gabriel as we walked around the show, but as soon as I saw her smiling face beaming at me as she walked towards us I changed my mind.

Maybe today I could just be Michelle. Not Michelle with a broken heart or Michelle whose baby died, or Michelle who is hoping and praying for a miracle. Just Michelle, a mum walking around the show having fun with her little boy and beautiful friend. I could tell Leah later and she would understand. Today I just needed to breathe.

It had rained heavily the night before so the three of us trudged through the mud visiting each stall and soaking up the sunshine. Preston loved meeting the local police officers and firemen. He climbed up with Leah and sat in the fire truck pressing buttons and pretending to be the driver. I took photos of them and watched as they had fun climbing around the truck. I was still feeling quite exhausted and was so grateful to have Leah there doing the climbing for me. She had no idea how I was feeling, but was just that kinda gal who loved to get in on the fun with Preston.

We headed to the local council display to find a huge garbage truck which Preston was so excited to sit in. Watching the garbage trucks collect our bins each week had been a major event in our house, with whoever was closest to Preston running to the front door to open it for him.

As we walked around the show I felt myself smiling. I was having such a lovely time and was so glad we came. After the garbage trucks we turned the corner and my brother-in-law Malcolm came into view. Malcolm and my step-sister Jess have three beautiful girls, Chloe, Libby and Kirsty. Having no daughters of my own I love getting my girl fix when we are all together.

I hoped that I could return the favour to uncle Mal whenever Preston was around. He worked for a local earth moving company and stood at the show in his cowboy hat, surrounded by huge earth-moving machines. Preston was so excited as uncle Mal lifted him up on to the biggest machine I've ever seen. I was so glad Mal was there. Preston could be quite shy around strangers but he was happy to climb up and sit on uncle Mal's lap. This part of our day was definitely a highlight for Preston.

We said goodbye to Mal and headed into the baby animal farm. Kids were running around from one animal pen to the other. Preston sat next to Leah and she put a baby rabbit in his lap. He looked up at me and gave me the biggest smile. My heart jumped.

He sat there for such a long time, holding on to the small bunny, with a look of love in his eyes. Every now and then Leah swapped animals for him. He sat so quietly while the others kids ran around us, in what seemed like total chaos. He was such a good boy, so quiet and patient. I hoped that one day if we were blessed with another baby, that he or she would have the same temperament. To me he was perfect.

We spent the rest of the day giving Preston the full show experience. We brought him two show bags and took a ride on the ferris wheel. As we reached the top of the ferris wheel Leah took a photo of Preston sitting on my lap. I held him tight and kissed his cheek as she clicked away.

I felt so grateful that I could hold him. So blessed that when things were bad I had this little miracle to hold tight and fill my heart with joy. I wondered how hard it must be for the mums who lose their first baby to miscarriage. I can only imagine how difficult it would be to have never held your own baby in your arms and not know if, or when, it would happen.

Preston had been my reason to get out of bed on so many occasions since losing our baby. Holding him in my arms brought so much peace to my heart. He was my miracle baby and being thankful for him, somehow made the pain I carried easier to bare. I'm not sure how I would have coped without this little guy to hold on to. As I sat on that ferris wheel watching thousands of people walk below us, my heart ached for every mum who was still waiting and hoping to one day hold on tight to a child of their own.

We headed out of the show and drove home. That afternoon I messaged Leah and thanked her for a beautiful day. I told her about our baby and how sad I had been. I said that it was so nice to be outside and we couldn't have picked a better friend to explore the show with. For the first time in a long time, I felt like I could breathe again.

# 22

## mother's day without my baby

Soon it was Mother's Day, and the grief hit me hard again. I could feel myself getting stressed leading up to it. I wasn't sure how I would feel celebrating being a mum without one of my babies in my arms. Usually Mother's Day is such a joyful time. The previous Mother's Day Jonathan and Preston took me into Sydney. We went out for lunch, then to the aquarium and we had ice cream at Circular Quay. It was a wonderful day and I loved every second of it.

This year was different. Leading up to it there was nothing planned. Jonathan and I were both exhausted and I think a little unsure of what emotions the day would bring. We celebrated with his mum a few days before so that Jonathan, Preston and I could have time together alone on Mother's Day, just the three of us.

The day came and I started to feel a little resentful that we didn't plan anything. Was Mother's Day not as important this year? Why was nothing planned? Why did things have to be so different? We went to church that morning. It was my turn on the roster to teach Kids Church. We made gifts for all the mums, we talked about how special mums are and prayed to thank God for the mums in our lives.

The kids also wrote down all the reasons they loved their mum. My heart was so heavy. If only I could celebrate Mother's Day pregnant this year.

I remembered back to the Mother's Day I was pregnant with Preston. It was too early to tell anyone. I sat in church pregnant and they asked all the mums and mums-to-be to put their hands up so they could hand out the gifts. I sat there quietly, smiling on the inside. Jonathan wasn't there, so as much as I wanted to jump up and yell out "I'm pregnant!" I had to hold it in.

This Mother's Day was very different. That joy I felt three short years ago was gone. I felt lost, hopeless and like a dark cloud was hovering over me. After church Preston fell asleep in the car so we grabbed some McDonald's on the way home. At this stage I was feeling a bit unimpressed and I think Jonathan could tell. He promised a fun afternoon once Preston woke up, and it was. The three of us went for a walk to the park and played for a while. Preston and I climbed up a big rock and sat together for our annual Mother's Day photo. My heart was still heavy but at least we were out doing something together. We went to an Italian restaurant for dinner and then out for ice cream. The Italian was a hit. Preston shovelled spaghetti bolognese into his mouth in such large quantities that people stopped as they walked past to tell us how adorable he was.

When we got home Jonathan and Preston gave me my gifts and a card. When I opened the card I felt the tears I had been holding down all day jump from my heart to my throat. The card read "To mummy, you are everything I could wish for in a mum! Thank you for always loving me, even when I do a poo in the shower!! Love Preston and Gabriel xoxo".

There it was, Gabriel's sweet name on my Mother's Day card. It filled my heart with joy and sadness all at the same time. We hadn't spoken about him in a couple of weeks. I was worried that Jonathan was starting to forget about him. This card showed me that Gabriel was just as real to him as he was to me. He was and always would be a part of our family. That card took the edge off the pain. It reminded me that on Mother's Day each year I could celebrate being a mum to all of my babies, not just the ones I held in my arms.

## 23

---

# when to try again?

Choosing the right time to try for another baby was such a big decision for us. In those first few weeks I was adamant that we would wait quite some time before trying again. I didn't want to replace Gabriel and I wanted to give him the respect he deserved. I wanted him to know how much his mummy and daddy loved him and that he held a special place in my heart and in our family.

I have friends who miscarried their first baby and tried again a month later. They felt the next baby helped with the healing process and found they were even more grateful for their child after what they had been through.

I also had other friends who waited a while to let their hearts mend a little. We have some friends who still can't even talk about the baby they lost and that's ok too. We are all so different. We all feel the pain in different ways and deal with the pain in our own way. There are no rules when it comes to grief, especially when it comes to losing a child.

My doctor told me to wait at least one cycle before trying for another baby. Even after waiting that short time I felt part of me was ready and part of me was not. I worried how I would feel with the next pregnancy test. Would it be the same as the last two? Would there be joy and elation or fear and anxiety? I wanted so badly for it to be a joyous occasion. I want my next pregnancy and baby to be enjoyed. I wanted for everyone close to us to be excited and not worried that something bad might happen.

I had so many feelings and worries to deal with. I didn't want to feel guilty. I didn't want people to look at me pregnant and think "wow she didn't wait long". I didn't want people to think that this baby would make everything better or that this baby was a replacement for Gabriel.

This baby would certainly help me to move forward but it wouldn't make everything better. It wouldn't take away the pain. To be honest I didn't want it to. But I knew that no matter what we decided we couldn't let what other people thought worry us. Nobody knows how much love I have for Gabriel. Nobody knows what I have been through to get to this point. I had to remind myself often that the people who love us will understand and be happy for us no matter what. I had to do what was best for me and my family.

Ultimately I believe that we don't really have a say in our children's birth dates. I think this was decided long ago. I knew that we would be waiting for as long or as little as it took. I knew that our baby would be here in God's perfect timing and I didn't want to rush that.

I think seeing Preston with Joseph helped me to be strong enough to start trying again. There's a two and a half year age gap between my brother Michael and I, and I love him so much. We had such a fun childhood together and I wanted the same for my babies. There's no doubt we wanted another baby but many things needed to be taken into consideration. The fear of miscarrying again was one of them.

I knew in my heart that our desire for another child totally outweighed the risk of losing another baby. If it were to happen again it would hurt so much, my heart would break all over again, but that couldn't stop me from trying. To not have another baby at all would hurt so much more, and I didn't believe that was God's plan for our family.

We waited a month for my cycle to return to normal and then made the decision to leave the conception of our next baby in God's hands.

I had no idea how I would feel to be pregnant again. Part of me wanted it so badly. Part of me was in a continual battle against fear and I was still so sad. I would often close my eyes and just picture Gabriel in my arms, asleep on my chest.

My heart was still in pieces, but what difference would another month or two months or six months or even a year make? I felt the desire to give Preston a sibling was much stronger than the desire to protect my heart from another loss, and so we tried again.

## 24

---

# pregnant

I took a deep breath. "This time will be different", I whispered to myself as I sat the positive pregnancy test back on the bathroom vanity. My heart ached. It seemed like only yesterday I was on my knees thanking God for my pregnancy with Gabriel. Yet so soon, here we were again. It had been three months since we lost our beautiful baby. I was excited to be pregnant again, but I was much more cautious than before. I didn't want to be scared. I needed to stay positive.

Jonathan and I made the decision that we wouldn't let fear take hold of us this pregnancy. Sure, there would be the usual concerns that every pregnant mum had, but I didn't want to be freaking out each day that my baby was gone or that I would miscarry.

I found a sympathetic ear in my friend Julia. I told her that in my heart I believed everything would be ok, I just had to get my head on the same page. She was so beautiful and helped me to stay positive in those early days and weeks. Whenever I started to worry she was always there for me. I really didn't expect anything would go wrong or that I would miscarry again. I was hoping the first 12 weeks would go quickly though, just to get to that "safe zone".

I rang and booked my midwife appointment and had a blood test to confirm the pregnancy. Everything was going well. I was nervous, but I truly believed that this baby was here to stay. This would be the baby that would remind me every day that God that delivers on His promises.

We started planning for the future again. I was five weeks pregnant when we bought a new car. Mine was falling apart and we needed something bigger for our growing family. It was an SUV and I loved driving it. Preston would always ask me to open the sunroof and remind me to close it whenever we arrived at our destination. I started to feel happy again. I felt that this pregnancy had made me feel even more grateful for my life and all I had. I still carried with me the heartache of losing Gabriel but I knew he was always with us. I knew that we would be together again one day.

This baby was due in February on my dad's birthday. I knew he would be so excited to share his birthday with his grandchild. I started thinking of ways to tell our family we were pregnant. Deciding when to tell them was also a big decision. Do we tell them early, so they can pray, or make them wait to make sure everything was ok?

I remember how hard it was to tell people that we lost our first baby, when they didn't even know we were pregnant. Rather than feel what we were feeling, there was mixed emotions. They seemed shocked that we were pregnant, but then sad that the baby was gone. I think if they had experienced the excitement that we did, when we first found out we were pregnant, then it might have made things easier for them and for us, to grieve afterwards.

This time around I was keen to tell a select few and ask them to pray for us. I had made a point of praying and giving thanks for this child. I didn't feel the need to go into battle and pray up a storm of protection each day. I felt like God had it all under control and that nothing could go wrong. After all, how much more could we take. It took enough strength to try again, let alone live through another miscarriage. I wasn't sure if my heart could take it, so I had no choice but to believe that everything would be ok.

# 25

five weeks

It was a sunny Thursday afternoon. I had spent the day with Preston. We went to playgroup in the morning, and spent the afternoon in the sunshine, walking around the block and stopping at every playground along the way.

It was a beautiful day. I was feeling so happy. Preston was at the stage where you could have long conversations with him. He was such an amazing little boy. As we walked along the footpath in the sunshine, I was thinking about what we had been through and the promise that was to come.

I had the life I always dreamed of, a loving husband, great house in a beautiful neighbourhood and a beautiful little boy. I was pregnant again and so excited to see Preston as a big brother. I had decided not to tell him this time until I was much further along. Not that I thought something would go wrong, I just couldn't put him through that again if it did, not so soon.

I watched as Preston sat down at the park and played in the garden for a while. The sunlight pierced through the trees as we sat in silence playing with the dirt. This day has lived on in my mind as one of the good ones. Maybe because we had nowhere else to be, or because I felt so much peace in this moment. Or perhaps this imprint in my memory has something to do with how quickly things can change, how quickly we can lose our peace.

That night I sat on our lounge in front of the heater watching the monitor and waiting for Preston to fall asleep. Jonathan was ordering car parts on eBay for our new car. Then all of a sudden I felt some cramping start. It came out of nowhere. I looked online and read that this was normal. I thought back to losing Gabriel and remembered I had light cramping for a couple of days before the heavy cramps started. This was different.

The cramping got much worse really quickly. I began to worry. This didn't feel normal. Something was wrong. My mind went into overdrive. Is it happening again? Surely not. Pray pray pray I thought. Or is it too late? There's no blood. It might be fine. I just need to relax and wait. Trust God. Have faith. Everything will be ok.

I considered cancelling my plans for the next day. We were going to a place called Featherdale Wildlife Park with my friends Christine and Brian and their son Ollie. Brian had organised it as a surprise for Christine because he had the day off work. He invited us along so that Preston and Ollie could see the Australian animals and feed the kangaroos together.

I really didn't want to cancel. It was going to be such a fun day and Preston had been talking about it all week. But should I rest? Should I tell Brian I'm unwell. Or is this just the pains that some women feel during these early weeks? Was this a good sign?

The next morning came and I decided to brave it. There was no blood and I was trying to stay positive. I considered telling them I was pregnant when we arrived, just in case something went wrong. I convinced myself that I was being paranoid and there was no need to worry. I packed Preston's lunch, got us both dressed and headed to our friends house. When we arrived, Preston told Christine and Ollie our plans for the day. They were so excited and ran around getting ready while Brian transferred Preston's car seat into his car.

Within half an hour the car seat was in and everyone was packed up ready to go. The cramping had gotten worse, so I excused myself to go to the bathroom quickly before we left. I sat down slowly and prayed as I peed, but it was way too late for that. I looked down to see the brightest red blood I had ever seen.

My heart hit my throat. Tears welled in my eyes.

My baby was gone.

## 26

---

# featherdale

I had a choice.

I could burst into tears and tell them what had happened. They could take the car seat back out of the car and cancel their plans. Then I could go home and cry for the rest of the day, or the rest of my life.

Or, I could take a deep breath and walk out of there like nothing had happened. I thought about Preston. He had already been through so much. He was only two years old. What would happen if he saw his mummy a mess again and was told there's no kangaroos today. This time would be different. I needed to protect him.

I messaged Jonathan. "Babe, I'm bleeding. I don't know why this is happening again. Please pray for me."

I wiped my face and looked in the bathroom mirror. "You can do this," I whispered. I took a deep breath and walked out of there like nothing had happened. I pushed every feeling right down and refused to let myself think about what was happening now or what had happened before. I could do that later. The world could stop later.

I was about to jump in the car when Jonathan rang. "What's

happening? Are you ok? What do you need? Are you going to the hospital?"

I told him that I was fine and that it was too late for the hospital. "Just pray for me to get through today. We can talk later my love. The kangaroos are waiting."

I sat in the car and we were on our way. My heart was ok for now. I think I was in shock. There was no fear or sadness. To be honest I didn't know how I felt. It was like I was on autopilot. I felt numb. There was a thick fog in my brain and I wanted it to stay. I just had to get through the day. I took two paracetamol for the cramping but my heart would have to wait.

As we pulled out of the street, Brian started talking to the GPS system in his car with his thick Maltese accent, "OK Google," he said. "Directions to Featherdale". The GPS system didn't understand a word he said and replied "Directions to Recreation Centre". I held in my smile. Brian pressed a button and tried again in frustration, but speaking louder only made his accent stronger "Directions to Featherdale" he said again loudly. I really hope the audio book can do his accent justice.

As Brian argued with the GPS system I thought about how life continues to move forward even when bad things happen. Here I was, sitting in my friend's car, with my heart in pieces, and nobody else knew what was going on.

Brian fighting with the GPS was actually hilarious, but I couldn't laugh for two reasons: one, I didn't want to disrespect my friend or his accent; and two, I was numb.

I felt totally removed from what was happening, but I also knew that no matter what happened in the next 24 hours or the next week, my life would continue to move forward and I would be ok. One day I would laugh again. Just not today.

I wasn't sure if I had some kind of divine protection around me, holding things together, or if I truly had shut off all emotions. We walked around the wildlife park watching Preston and Ollie chase the kangaroos. We even had a brush with fame, bumping in to Kelly Rowland and her son Titan. She was in Australia at the time filming *The Voice*. There's nothing like seeing a gorgeous superstar and her cute kid to take your mind off things. It was so surreal for me. I was actually pregnant with Preston at the same time Kelly was pregnant with her little boy. They were both born in November 2014. To see them playing around the kangaroos together was so precious. I had no idea what Kelly's story was, or if she had ever experienced what I was going through at that moment. But she seemed to be such a beautiful mum to her little boy. I'm so glad I got to witness that. I'm so glad that she was there that day to distract me from my heartache.

The boys were all so excited, especially when the animals came up to eat from their little hands. I looked at Preston and knew that I had made the right decision to continue our day as planned. Then and there I decided that I wouldn't cry in front of him this time. I wasn't sure his sensitive little heart could take it again.

Like I mentioned before, I think it's important to show our emotions in front of our kids. It's good for them to see us come through the storm. Everyone's circumstance is different. During my first miscarriage Preston saw me cry on and off for weeks. I literally couldn't hold it in. The second time around I knew that Preston would sense something was wrong, I just decided not to let him see the worst of it.

We were only at the Wildlife Park for a couple of hours. The pain killers weren't doing much for the cramping and I was secretly hoping that one of the boys would need a nap soon so we could go home. It wasn't so much that I was holding back tears or fighting emotions. I wasn't at all. I was just in a lot of pain and totally exhausted. I wanted to lay down on the lounge and sleep for as long as it took for the pain to go away.

When we got back to Christine and Brian's house they asked if I wanted to stay for the afternoon. I used Preston's nap time as an excuse to leave. When we got home I actually decided to keep Preston awake. If he didn't nap, then he would go to bed earlier and have a good night sleep, which is what we both needed.

We spent the afternoon on the lounge, watching television, surrounded by a messy house.

I started to worry a little. Why wasn't I crying? Where were all the emotions I felt last time? Was I stronger this time around? To me that was doubtful. Was I numb inside because this could actually be serious? Was I refusing to face the fact that there could be a medical issue stopping me from carrying a baby? My mind began to race again.

Every now and then I'd start to think about Gabriel, and then just before the flood of emotions came, I would stop and think about something else. I couldn't believe how easy it was to stop those thoughts. Maybe I did it for Preston. Maybe seeing him so upset a few months ago helped me to hold it in. I had no idea what to do or what to think. I felt nothing, I felt empty.

# 27

---

## aunty peta, what you doing?

I decided to message my sister-in-law Peta and asked her to pray for me. I told her I had miscarried again, but asked her not to tell anyone. She waited for her kids to wake up from their naps, packed them in the car along with a stir-fry for dinner, some savoury muffins and a pineapple.

She asked if I wanted her to leave Joseph at home with Rob, just in case a baby was too much for my heart to deal with. I told her to bring both kids. They would be a good distraction. I knew there was no way I could be upset in front of Preston again so they might as well come. I still wasn't sure how I felt about anything.

She arrived and the boys played. Every now and then, when Preston wasn't around us I would mention something about the week's events to fill her in. I told her about my doctors appointment, the blood tests, and then miscarrying at the Wildlife Park. We went through the motions, feeding the boys dinner and bathing them. Jonathan was still at work so it was nice to have company. I think having them there helped to keep the heartbreaking reality out of my head and protect my heart. I began to wonder, who was I really protecting, Preston or myself?

Before Peta left to go home, the boys were playing in our toy room. She came over and hugged me so tight. She began to whisper a prayer in my ear and placed her hand on my stomach. She prayed for my heart, she prayed for the Lord's comfort, she prayed against fear, and then we heard a little voice from underneath us say "Aunty Peta, what you doing?"

It was Preston, of course, my curious bright-eyed boy. "Giving mummy a cuddle" she answered. Preston immediately climbed up onto the lounge in between us to get in on the action. I sat on the lounge in a three-way-hug with two of my favourite people and still no tears. I couldn't believe it. A heartfelt prayer, a super long hug and my beautiful boy joining in, but somehow the tears didn't flow.

When Jonathan got home Preston was in bed asleep. He hugged me and we sat on the lounge. There really wasn't much to say. I explained that it mustn't have hit me yet. That I was just going through the motions, waiting to feel something, but blocking it all out at the same time.

Jonathan said he felt numb. He didn't have words. He didn't know what to say.

We were both in this strange place where we really didn't think that it would ever happen to us again. We didn't think that losing another baby was part of our story, and neither of us were ready to face the truth that our second beautiful baby was gone.

# music heals the soul

Twenty-four hours later and I was still feeling numb and exhausted. I was in great physical pain and felt like my mind was covered by a mental fog. I cancelled all of our weekend plans. I felt there was no need to be a hero and I wanted to stay in bed.

On Sunday Jonathan went to work, and Preston and I spent the day in our pyjamas. I made him breakfast, we played with cars, lego and watched some tv. I didn't feel like I was fighting back tears, I just felt like I couldn't feel anything. I wasn't angry or upset, I wasn't anything. It was so completely different this time around, so surreal.

I began to feel guilty. How must it look to my baby that his mum wasn't even crying?

Would my baby wonder why I hadn't shed even one tear, or wonder if I was even thinking about him? I was so confused. Why couldn't I grieve this baby the same way I had grieved Gabriel? I didn't even feel like I was holding in tears. I didn't want to cry or be sad. I struggled to think about the future. I began to think that there was something wrong with me.

By Sunday night I knew that something had to give. When

Jonathan got home from work we sat on the lounge to watch *The Voice* together. One of the contestants, Judah Kelly, sang 'Iris', a song by the Goo Goo Dolls.

Then it happened.

He sang the first line, "And I'd give up forever to touch you" and I burst into tears. I cried and cried and cried until I couldn't breathe. The flood gates had opened. I couldn't hold it in. This time was supposed to be different. This was supposed to be my rainbow baby, the one who would bring light back into our family. I loved this baby and I didn't want to go through this again. In this moment, listening to this song, reality hit me hard and I felt the devastation flow through my body.

I thought about Gabriel and all the things I had done to make sure he had a place in our family. I spent so much time thinking about him and making sure that he would be loved and remembered always. As the song played I thought about this baby. He needed a name, he needed a Christmas bauble, he needed to know that his mum and dad loved him so much. My heart felt crushed all over again.

I tried a few deep breaths to stop the tears but it didn't work. There was no stopping it. Jonathan moved closer on the lounge. He put his arm around me and closed his eyes. He was praying. I could tell. Slowly but surely I stopped crying and started breathing again. What a release. It had only been two days but it seemed like I had been holding those tears in for a lifetime.

About 20 minutes later Judah came back on the stage for his second song. They announced that he would be singing Hallelujah by Leonard Cohen. Jonathan looked at me and said "Are you going to be alright with this babe?" I smiled.

The answer was no. I heard him slowly sing those beautiful words over and over again "hallelujah, hallelujah, hallelujah". More tears, but this time different. This time with his words I could actually feel the love of Jesus flow through my body. It wasn't just Jono holding me close, my Lord, my saviour was in the room.

Bits and pieces from different bible verses started flooding into my mind all mixed up together, "be not afraid, I am your God, I will carry you. When you pass through the waters I will be with you. When you walk through the fire you will not be burned. Cast all your cares on me. The Lord is near the broken-hearted. He saves those crushed in spirit. He hears their cries and saves them. Take heart I have overcome the world".

Music for my ears and words for my soul. In the final chapter of this book I have written a few bible verses that have helped me through the darkest days of my life. I still to this day read over them to fill me with God's love, peace and comfort.

The next day I pulled myself together again for Preston. I had made an appointment with our family GP, Dr Trang. I love our doctor. She's so sweet and kind and has been a wonderful support for our family. She had seen me at my worst shortly after I miscarried Gabriel and held my hand as I cried at her desk.

This time I sat across from her again, and I told her we had lost another baby. Much different to last time, I sat in silence for a while. No tears, just silence. I asked if she could do some tests, or if there was anything I could be doing wrong? She looked at me with compassion. "Michelle, you've done nothing wrong. It's something we can't explain. If it happens again I will send you to a specialist."

She took my hand again and said "Are you ok?" I smiled a fake smile, looked at Preston playing with his toy cars and shook my head. "No," my voice broke. I told her I wasn't ok, but I was going to do things differently this time and not cry in front of Preston. She understood, but I could tell she was concerned. She asked if Jonathan would be at home with me this week and booked me in to see her a week later for a follow up.

Before we drove home I sat in my car and made some calls to book in an ultrasound and a blood test for later that week. I needed to make sure the miscarriage completed naturally. On the way home we stopped for some groceries and the cramping started again. It was a harsh reminder that my body was not ready for too much movement. I was trying to be strong for my boy, but I needed to rest. I needed some time to grieve again. My body had failed me. My baby was gone, and the plans we had for our family had fallen through, again.

## 29

---

# sisterhood

It was 7am. I laid in bed looking out into the small courtyard through our French doors. I could hear Preston and Jonathan making pancakes in the kitchen. I wanted to get up and join them but I couldn't move. I was physically and emotionally exhausted. I was sad, but at the same time I was tired of being sad. I was tired of worrying about the future, tired of being in a situation that I desperately didn't want to be in. In that moment I felt such heaviness, pushing my body down into the mattress. Losing our second baby had taken my anxiety to another level. Our situation was becoming overwhelming, and I could feel that I had lost my peace.

I wanted to fast forward. I wanted to close my eyes and be out of the darkness, far from this place of fear and uncertainty. I wanted to be in a happier place, where my broken heart was a distant memory. I stared out the window and longed for some peace. I'm not sure how long I laid there, feeling so anxious, but all of a sudden I knew where I needed to be. On Thursday mornings I sometimes visited the Sisterhood service at our local Hillsong Church. It was a special service just for women, that I loved to attend whenever I could. I wasn't sure exactly why, but I knew that's where I needed to be.

I got out of bed and shuffled along the cold tiles, down the hallway, into the kitchen.

"Berry pancakes mummy!" said Preston all excited, followed by "it's already morning you know?"

I smiled and kissed his forehead. Jonathan put down the spatula and wrapped his arms around me. My love, my safe place. How I longed to stay there in his arms all day, but I knew I had somewhere else to be. I ate breakfast with my boys and headed to church. As hard as it was to get out of my dressing gown and into some real clothes, a good dose of Sisterhood was exactly what I needed. There's a lot to say about the power of women coming together for a purpose. Girls, mothers, daughters, friends, all coming together to grow their faith, and to love and support one another. Whilst nobody there would know about our babies, they were all such lovely, kind and compassionate women to be around. I knew I was heading into a safe place.

I parked my car and walked towards the church. Usually whenever I visited I would invite a friend to come along with me, but today was different. For some reason it seemed right to come alone. I walked through the doors and received a hug from the ladies on the welcome team. I saw my friend Sharon across the room. She was pregnant, gorgeous and glowing. She saw me and smiled her beautiful smile.

I've known Shaz for about ten years. She's such an amazing mum. This was her second baby and I was so happy for her. She made such gorgeous children and I loved watching her family grow. We didn't see each other very often, but when I did see her, Shaz always made me feel so loved. She's always had this heavenly glow about her, a glow I loved to be around. When she saw me arrive, Shaz walked straight over and wrapped her arms around me. I felt her pregnant belly press up against me. I tried not to think about the empty womb beneath my jumper, I tried not to think about my babies, or my broken heart, because despite our circumstances, it was a hug that filled me with so much peace. I felt at home. Love conquers all.

"It's so good to see you, I'm so glad you're here," she said as we hugged.

I swallowed my tears and smiled "me too".

I didn't want to cry. I didn't feel like talking about my broken heart. I just wanted to be there, in that moment. I wanted to escape the darkness, I needed to find my peace. We walked into the auditorium and sat down. The worship music started playing and instantly I felt some heaviness lift from me. I looked over at Shaz, standing in the front row with both her arms up in the air as she sang and praised the Lord for His goodness. I wondered if one day that would be me again. Pregnant and praising the Lord with all my heart and all my soul. I took a deep breath and closed my eyes. I felt my mind begin to clear. I felt like I could breathe again. Maybe just for now, but it was nice to breathe.

After worship we took our seats and Pastor Bobbie Houston began to give her message. She spoke about Abigail, a woman in the bible who was a peacemaker, and how brave she was despite the challenge she faced. As Pastor Bobbie shared the story of Abigail, I felt like she was speaking to my heart. She spoke about peace being the intent of God in our lives. She said that no matter what our circumstances, God has a plan of divine intervention for us, a plan for peace just like He did for Abigail. My story and my circumstance was very different to Abigail's, but I still felt, that just like her, I would have to fight for my peace. I needed to be strong and not let go of the promise. I

97

needed to trust God that His intent for me and my family was one of peace and joy, and I couldn't settle for anything less.

I drove home from church with tears running down my face. I wondered if I was brave enough. I wondered if I had what it takes. I wondered how long I would still feel this way, and I prayed that one day, once all my tears had finished, that I would finally find my peace.

*30*

# my little raphie

It wasn't long before I felt that longing to name our baby. As much as I hated the thought of having to name another child that I couldn't hold in my arms, I knew that we had to do it. There would be no peace in my heart while our baby was in heaven without a name.

I thought back to our list when we named Gabriel, and how much the meaning of his name meant to us. God is my strength, bringer of light. I had leant on God's strength so much to get me through the first loss and I felt His strength even more now to get me through again.

I remembered we liked the name Raphie. It means God has healed. Then for the middle name either Jon for a boy, like Preston after his daddy, or Joan for a girl after my nan. Because we didn't know the gender of this baby we stuck with the letter J and chose the middle name Jay, which means to rejoice.

Raphie Jay – God has healed, to rejoice.

To us the name is perfect. I believe that its meaning is prophetic. We know God is our healer. We are declaring that God has already healed, because we know that He will. Then 'to rejoice' is also a sign of things to come. We know that God will send us a baby sibling for Preston when the time is right, and we know that the day we see Gabriel and Raphie in heaven we will rejoice, for all of eternity.

The weeks following, I started to think a lot about Raphie and pray for him. For some reason the image of a boy came more clearly in my mind than a girl. But that may be because I am used to having a little boy under my feet. I wondered what life would be like if we had Gabriel and Raphie here with us too.

As I prayed and thought about him I felt like Raphie would have been a mummy's boy. Was this God giving me a picture of my children? Was this His way of keeping them as part of our family? I hoped so. Those babies were so real to me, and through God I felt I could continue a connection with them until we are all together once more.

When I talk about this baby I always call him "My little Raphie". My youngest child so far, a beautiful and perfect creation from God. Another baby that my heart would always ache for, an ache that will forever remind me of what I have lost, but would also remind me of how strong I can be with God on my side.

It felt bitter sweet sending a little brother or sister up to heaven for Gabriel. I was pleased that they would always be together. Just like I wanted a sibling for Preston, I also wanted my kids in heaven to have someone close to them. I knew they wouldn't be alone.

My cousin Belinda lost her little girl Harper about six months before we lost Gabriel. Her experience was one of great heartbreak and courage, but that is her story to tell. We both only have brothers, so Belinda has always been like a sister to me. We often speak about the three of our babies growing up together just like we did.

God often gives me visions of them, playing together, singing and dancing. They are so close in age that they are almost like triplets.

Whenever I see them they are full of so much joy. While my heart aches for them now, I know that there are no tears in heaven, only love, peace and joy. I know that one day, thanks to our faith we will all feel that joy together.

## 31

---

# rejoice

Raphie's middle name ended up being a very important part of my journey. As I mentioned, Jay means to rejoice. A few days after my miscarriage I was in bed trying to sleep and I became overwhelmed with grief.

Jonathan was out in the lounge room and heard me crying. He came in and sat with me. I buried my head in his jumper and sobbed my heart out.

There it was. The darkness in my mind and heart, back again. I knew it well. This time was different though. I had already been through the fire with Gabriel. God had literally carried me out of the darkest time in my life. This time I knew He would do it again. I just had to feel it. I felt like I had to let myself cry all the tears. I needed to grieve so that I could open my heart for God's healing.

Jonathan didn't say anything. My heart ached for him too. The person I loved most on this earth couldn't put into words the grief he was feeling. He was so numb and so shocked that we were going through this again that he couldn't speak.

I looked at him with tears running down my face. "Are you going to say something?" I whispered. He looked at me and took a deep breath. "I'm so sorry babe," he said "I just don't know what to say." We hugged a while longer and I laid down to try and sleep. Jonathan went back out to the lounge room.

I knew I wouldn't be able to sleep. My heart was in pieces. I was full of fear. I was scared to be alone with my thoughts and my feelings. I felt like every ounce of hope I had was crushed. I opened my bible and prayed "What about you Lord?" I whispered. "Are you going to say something?"

I flicked my bible open to a random page and found Psalm 130:5.

*I wait for the Lord, my soul waits, and in His word I do hope.*

My heart skipped a beat. I whispered it over and over again. I wait for the Lord, my soul waits and in His word I do hope.

My chest began to feel heavy and I knew I needed more. I jumped online and sent that verse to a few friends from my church. Then it happened. God came in the room.

My friends could see that me sending this verse was a cry for help. I didn't have the words to send them. The bible verse was all I could manage to send along with a cry face emoji.

The first thing they did was send me a photo of Jesus with his arm stretched out and a bible verse: I will strengthen you and help you; I will uphold you with my righteous right hand (Isaiah 41:10). Then they told me that nothing they could say would take away the pain I was feeling. So back and forth we went sending bible verses and prayers.

In our prayers we thanked God for his love and comfort and for always being there in our darkest hour. We thanked Him for looking after our babies in heaven and for all the good things to come. My friends spoke life into me. They told me they loved me and that I was an amazing mum. One couple had lost a baby themselves and shared

103

their heartbreak with me. They told me that God's army was with us, and they were all standing with me and Jonathan.

Then came the breakthrough. I decided to share the name of our baby with our friends and the reason we chose Raphie Jay – God has healed, to rejoice. They sent me a screenshot of a conversation they had with another friend earlier that evening. In that message they had told this friend that God kept giving them the word "Rejoice!"

My heart stopped again. God had spoken. He had spoken the meaning of the middle name of my precious baby to a friend who he knew I would turn to for help later that night. God could see me. God knew my pain. God cries when we cry and He smiles when we smile. He dances when we dance. He knows the song in our hearts.

All of a sudden our conversation was based on this word from God. Rejoice, Rejoice, Rejoice! We spoke about how wonderful it will be the day God blesses us with a baby. God spoke to me that night. He told me that we would rejoice, he said that I would dance for Him. I began making declarations about God turning our mourning into dancing.

I had also sent that verse to my friend Ashleigh. She replied with two simple words, "Trust Him" and sent me a photo of Psalm 139 from her bible. You have searched me Lord and you know me. You know when I sit and when I rise, you perceive my thoughts from afar. You discern my going out and my lying down; you are familiar with all my ways.

God was telling me that he knows my heart. He knows the grief I feel. He knows how much I love my babies and how much I want another baby. He knows what a good big brother Preston will be. He knows how much my family means to me. He loves me so much, and I needed to trust Him.

It was after midnight and God had turned my darkest hour into one where my heart was so full of love it could burst. I was thinking about the songs that helped me earlier that week. The song Hallelujah really spoke to me. As I laid in bed I looked up the meaning of the word and it said: "God be praised – uttered in worship or as an expression of rejoicing. An utterance of the word 'hallelujah' as an expression of worship or rejoicing."

There it was again, the word rejoice. I was quickly being filled with hope. I knew in my heart that we would rejoice. I just had to wait and trust in God that this day would come, and trust in His timing.

# dance mummy dance

One of the things God said to me as I cried to Him that night, I will never forget. "You will dance for me again." In those times when I was feeling my worst, it was so hard to picture myself dancing, especially the type of dancing I knew the Lord meant. There is a verse in the bible which says "…and David danced before the Lord with all his might". Every time I read it I picture my little niece Chloe, dancing at a Christmas concert years ago. She would have only been about three-years-old. She was dancing with so much force in every movement, and so much joy in her heart.

When God spoke those words to me I knew he meant that there would be joy in my house again. I just didn't realise how soon it would happen. The next night I put on some worship music while I was cooking dinner. Preston calls it "Jesus music". I love playing worship songs in our house. There is power in these songs to calm you down or lift you up, whatever the case may be. It certainly makes things calmer in our home. Whenever the music plays Preston is happy to play with his toys and listen to the music while I cook dinner.

That night, as I stirred the curry on the stove, Preston came into the kitchen. He was smiling ear to ear. An upbeat worship song had just come on. He started dancing under my feet. "Dance mummy dance," he said excitedly. "It's Jesus!" I loved watching this kid dance. It always filled me with joy. I put the lid on the saucepan and started dancing around the kitchen with him. What a release. I had tears in my eyes. We were singing and dancing together. I felt so much heaviness released from my heart. I felt blessed. I felt loved and I felt so happy. This was a beautiful memory. One that I will never forget.

I whispered "thank you" as we danced. I was thanking God for the beautiful child in front of me. Thanking Him for His peace and joy. Thanking Him that He was right, I would dance for Him again. My heart was still aching, but it was also full of love. As we danced around the kitchen all of a sudden we heard Jonathan's car pull into the driveway. Preston ran into his toy room to hide from daddy, a nightly occurrence where he would hide in exactly the same spot every time and wait for Jonathan to find him.

When Jonathan came in and found him, Preston ran to his toy box and grabbed a few musical instruments. He gave Jono the bongo drums and me the keyboard. He then rolled out his floor keyboard and started dancing on the giant keys to make music. It was so cute. Jonathan and I looked at each other and we both smiled. I could tell what he was thinking. No matter what happens we would always have each other and we will always come through the fire, no matter how much it hurt. We turned the worship music up and all started playing our instruments and dancing together in the toy room.

The next few nights, instigated by Preston, the three of us would dance and play instruments to worship music. I can't explain the feeling in my heart each time. I often have to remind myself that God loves me even more than I love Preston. It's hard to believe but it's true. We are His children and He loves us more than we love our own. It's such a perfect love. One that will reach in and pull us out of the darkness back into the light, time and time again.

It's the *Agape* love, an ancient Greek term referring to the highest form of love, and the most selfless love that we receive from the Lord. This love that had me dancing around the room, full of thanks and joy and love despite my broken heart. It doesn't matter how broken it is or how sad I felt, I knew that God would hold every piece of my heart together for as long as I needed Him to. It's for that reason that I will always dance for Him. No matter what my circumstance.

For some, it might be hard to imagine how I could possibly dance around the house so soon after losing Raphie. I know it definitely wouldn't be possible without my faith. It's so hard to put into words the affect our faith can have on our lives especially when we feel like we are walking through the fire. My heart still aches for Gabriel and Raphie, every single day, but I know that my babies are dancing around the feet of Jesus in heaven, just like Preston does in my kitchen.

## 33

# for such a time as this

There are times in our lives when we have no choice but to be brave, even when the world has fallen out from underneath us. As wives, as mums, as women, we can face the most heartbreaking situations and still find the strength, guts and courage to keep moving forward, whether it's one minute, one day or one hour at a time. After we lost our babies there were times when I felt so broken that I knew I needed time, time to be still, to feel the hurt and to grieve what I had lost. There were times that I was so full of fear of what the future would hold, and times that I had to draw strength from God just to get out of bed, to be strong and to move forward for my family.

There have been so many stories written throughout history, detailing just how strong and courageous women can be. One of my favourites, is the story of a Jewish woman named Esther in the Bible. She lived in Persia, married a King, and risked her own life to save her people. Esther's cousin Mordecai sent word to her that God had put her in this position for a reason. She was put there for *"such a time as this"*. I still remember the first time I heard this story. I was a new Christian, and my amazing Pastor at the time, Jill Bell, stood up at a women's event to share this story about a beautiful queen who drew her courage from the Lord, to save her people. In that moment I realised just how strong and brave I could be with God on my side, and I've never forgotten it.

There are times in our lives when God places us somewhere for a reason, and makes us stronger than we ever imagined we could be. Even when bad things happen it's not God who does the bad things to us, He loves us too much for that. The bible says that all things work for good for those who love the Lord. I feel now, more than ever, that I am living proof of that.

In the days after we lost Raphie, I knew that if I wanted to survive the aftermath of this miscarriage, then I would need to press in even deeper to God. I watched so much online preaching, and read my bible whenever I had the chance. I kept my head in the Psalms. They helped me to cry, and gave me hope of what was to come. I could feel myself getting closer to God. I started to hear his voice much clearer, and so many times He spoke to me through other people.

There's a pastor in Queensland, Australia, called Ben Hughes who preaches online and prays each day in live Facebook posts. Sometimes he prays for people who were watching online and gave them words of encouragement over their lives. One day he was preaching, and for some reason I just kept thinking, 'say my name' as he spoke. Maybe it was my recent encounter with Kelly Rowland, but her song even started bouncing around in my head, "*say my name, say my name*". He was just preaching that day and didn't give any prophetic words for his online listeners, but, all of a sudden with 40 seconds of his live feed to go, (I know this because I watched it back again), he stopped what he was saying, and said "Michelle". Nothing else. No prayer or prophetic words, just "Michelle" and then he kept talking.

I couldn't believe it. My name. Just my name. It made me think.

God knows my name. He knew it long before my parents did. He sees me. He wants me to know that he hears every thought and feels every feeling that I am feeling. My God is here with me. I was in this situation for a reason and I was determined to find out what that was.

Also that week Jonathan and I watched the movie War Room together. It was about a woman who used the power of prayer to save her marriage and her family. It was amazing and perfect timing.

There's a lot to say about the power of prayer, and the people who devote their lives to praying for others, and helping people to find strength in their darkest hour. A lovely couple named Pat and Jim, who were connected to our church, ran a healing ministry, and invited me to meet with them for some prayer. They prayed for me and filled me with so much hope. They gave me confidence that everything would be ok. Sometimes you just need people around you who will speak life and hope and positivity into your world. Our words and thoughts are so powerful and can have such a big impact on our journey.

I found that looking to God for comfort and peace and knowing that He is in control, helped remove the anxiety and stress out of the situation. I know that my next baby's birthday has already been decided. I know that no amount of worry is going to change things. I just had to trust in God.

If you have a medical condition that limits your chance to have a baby please don't think I'm saying that you should ignore all medical advice and just pray. There is certainly room for both. Prayer can enhance our healing journey in so many ways, whether it's supernatural healing or God holding our hand and giving us strength through treatments and procedures.

As I began to draw on God's strength I also started to fear that people might think losing Raphie wasn't as sad for me as losing

Gabriel. That's not true. They are both my babies and I love them so much. My heart felt the same grief and shock and sadness, but this time I truly felt God's hands holding my heart together. I know that there are scars, but if we let God heal those scars then we grow even stronger.

When we lost our babies we had a whole church praying for us. One Sunday our leaders anointed me with oil and prayed for my body and my broken heart. I had tears in my eyes as I felt my heart strengthen with every prayer.

Not long after we experienced our second miscarriage, this book suddenly came to life. I had started writing everything down after we lost Gabriel, but since losing Raphie the words began to flow out on to the page like a river. My hope is that this book would help as many parents as possible, who have been through this grief themselves. If I have lived through this to get closer to God and to help other people through their darkness, then I can't argue with that. God spoke to me that week. I found my strength in Him. He stuck closer to me than I ever thought possible to get me through it, and I am so grateful for that.

I don't know the big picture. I don't know why it had to hurt so much, but I do know that God has brought me here, 'for such a time as this'.

## 34

## my heart aches for you

I climbed into bed, freezing cold, and covered myself in blankets. Jonathan was at work and Preston was asleep, so I decided to take a look back through my journal. I wanted to read about my babies, I needed to look back over our journey and see how far we had come. I flicked open and started reading. How did this happen? How did my story change so much, and so quickly? I flicked back to before we had our first miscarriage, to see the types of things I was writing about a few short months ago.

I came across one page in particular and I froze. I couldn't remember writing it. I couldn't remember thinking anything of it at the time, but now looking back, the words pierced my heart. I felt overcome with shock, joy and sadness all at once. I must have prayed and asked God to speak to me. This is what He said:

*"Whatever comes against you, comes against me"*

*"I'm not going anywhere"*

*"I know what's ahead for you.*

*"I will hold you, catch you, carry you and be beside you"*

*"You are the apple of my eye."*

When I read this, after all we had been through, I felt so sad, but at the same time I felt so grateful, so loved, so protected. They say that being a Christian doesn't mean the storms won't come, it means that God will stand beside you when they do. This was an example where God had warned me that a storm was coming and promised to be with me through it all.

When I wrote these words I had no idea what was ahead for us. I felt so sad to think about how clueless I was back then, thinking it would be easy to just fall pregnant and have another baby. At the same time I felt so grateful that God was with me and that He was prepared for what was coming.

I flicked forward to the pages I wrote after losing Gabriel. I had drawn a picture of an image God had shown me of a red heart in pieces with cracks through it, some bigger than others. There were two big hands holding the heart together. After we lost Raphie, He showed me the same heart but with silver running through all the cracks, like liquid titanium filling all the gaps and gluing my heart back together. The silver had this Holy glow about it too, like the Holy Spirit had poured it in there to strengthen my heart.

We all have scars, emotional scars that are so bad only God can heal them. I know many people would say that once something is cracked or broken, it can never be repaired back to how it was. While I agree that a broken heart is never going to be how it was before, I also believe that the choices we make can decide if our hearts end up stronger or more fragile, after they are broken.

God showed me the titanium heart because He knew that if I held on tight to my faith and His word, that I would come out of this with a heart that was even stronger than it was before. As mums we feel those cracks so often and we have to dig deep to find that strength.

God can help us do that. Recently I was praying and God showed me the titanium melting away and those cracks in my heart being filled instead with the blood of Christ. Titanium will melt when the temperature reaches 1668 degrees celsius. I feel like the blood of Christ can withstand so much more than that. We saw it when Jesus died for us on the cross.

Doctors who have studied the description of the crucifixion, say the pain Jesus endured would have been beyond excruciating. The word excruciating actually means "out of the cross." The word comes from *Latin* excruciare, from cruciare, or to crucify. It means unbearably painful, or extreme agony. Jesus experienced the worst pain anyone could feel. It is because of the cross, that we know how much we are loved, and we can have hope in Christ's love no matter what circumstance or storm we face.

Also on the pages in my diary I noticed a few times that I had written *My heart aches for you*. At first I didn't understand what this meant, I thought perhaps the Lord's heart was aching because He wanted to be closer to me. Now that I have two babies in heaven I totally understand what it means for your heart to ache for a child. My heart aches for Gabriel and Raphie every single day. What I wouldn't give to hold my babies, to talk to them, to hear their voices, to feel them against my chest and to feel the love between us. God feels the same when it comes to me and you.

As I closed my journal I realised that really, it's all about love. Once I finally understood the depth of love that God has for me as His child, then I could rest in that love. I could find true peace and I could rest in His arms because He would take care of everything. There is nothing worse than losing a child. My heart is still broken, but it has also strengthened with every day, every hour, every moment that I have survived without them, and I'm so grateful for that.

## 35

## the month of may

I wrote the chapters in this book as they happened, so you will probably notice a range of emotions through the ups and downs I experienced on this journey. There were times when I felt strong, hopeful, positive and grateful, and times when I felt disheartened, broken, lost, hopeless, fearful and beaten.

After our second miscarriage the decision to keep trying, without taking a break in between, was based again on Preston. I had seen him with other babies and I had heard his prayers asking for Jesus to send us a new baby. I wanted him to be a big brother so much and to know what it felt like to have a sibling by your side as your best friend. With this in mind we kept trying. We prayed and trusted in God that His plans for our family were better than ours. We believed that the birthday of our baby was already written, so there was nothing we could do to rush that.

One thing we never had a problem doing was falling pregnant. I guess this made the decision to try again a big one. With each miscarriage came a new level of exhaustion and heartache. Knowing that we would most-probably fall pregnant again, meant that if we were to miscarry, it could be very soon. This took our trust in God to a whole new level. It was like we were trusting Him that everything would be ok, but also trusting Him that if things didn't work out, our hearts would survive another crushing so soon.

It was July and I had already had two miscarriages. I wasn't sure how much more I could take, but I knew that I couldn't give up. I knew that God wasn't surprised by what we had been through. He knew about everything before it happened and He stood by me through it all. I had to trust Him. I had to listen to Him and stay close to Him. It was the only way to make this work.

Each time we lost a child Dr Trang told us to wait one cycle before trying again. So we did. In a way that month of waiting felt like a lifetime, but somehow it also felt like no time at all. After losing Raphie I spent time with God in prayer. I wanted to hear from Him. I needed to know what He wanted. If He wanted us to wait or to keep trying. One day when I was praying I couldn't get a song out of my head. I knew it was from God. The song was *My Girl*, by the Temptations. For those who aren't familiar with the lyrics of the song, it says:

*"I've got sunshine on a cloudy day*
*When it's cold outside*
*I've got the month of May"*

If this was a Hollywood movie you could presume that I was going to have a baby in May. Only time would tell. Perhaps it was just God promising me that there would be sunshine again, perhaps He was reminding me that He was my sunshine on a rainy day, or maybe all of the above.

All I knew was that a May baby meant I would be pregnant the very next month after losing Raphie. So we handed our broken hearts over to God and we tried again.

# poppy louis

It was the day before my pop's funeral, when I started feeling sick to my stomach. It was the same sickness I had felt so many times before. My anxiety gut was back.

My heart sank. I hadn't had a "vomit attack" for more than six months. It had been so long that I was sure I had been healed and that dreadful season was behind me. But sure enough, I spent this particular Monday night on the bathroom floor. Vomiting every half an hour or so. No sleep, bad nausea and intense stomach pain.

My dad and step mum were staying the night. We were all so sad about my pop, but this added an extra dimension to our sadness. As much as they had been there for us through everything, they had never seen me so sick. I could tell they were worried. Whenever we were sick as kids my dad would always say that he wished he could take the pain away, so he could be sick instead of us. Thirty years later and nothing had changed. Between our tears for Pop, and my constant vomiting, I don't think any of us got much sleep that night.

The vomiting stopped at about 8am. I got dressed and drove for over an hour to the funeral. It was a beautiful service. A great tribute to a man who had sacrificed so much for his family. Poppy Louis had moved here from Malta with my nan in 1948 with their two children. Once settled in Australia they had five more children, including my dad. Pop spent his life working as a mechanic to provide for his family. He was a man of faith, a man of few words, but he was always so full of pride for his grandchildren.

When I became a journalist I used to send Nan and Pop cuttings from the newspaper with some of my favourite columns and articles. There was one in particular that Pop must have loved because he had it stuck up on his bedroom wall for many years. He was 96 years old when he passed away. He was a dedicated Catholic who went to church every week of his life without fail.

I was in a fair bit of pain all day at the funeral. I presumed it was muscular pain from a long night of vomiting. I felt weak and exhausted. But I wanted to be there for my dad and for Pop. I didn't want to miss my last chance to say goodbye. My brother Michael arrived and sat with me. I hugged him tight and felt so grateful that he was there.

I hobbled up to the altar in the church to give my reading. My heart was heavy, my stomach was aching and I was so fearful that my vomiting attacks were back. When I sat back in my seat I looked at the coffin and thought to myself, "You're in heaven now Poppy. You have all the answers, what is to become of me? What are God's plans for my family?"

I could feel the pain in my stomach. The freedom I had felt from not being sick for six months was slipping away. I felt lost and confused. We had put off trying for a baby before because I was too sick last year. Should we wait again, or keep trying? I now had these vomiting attacks to add to the possibility of another miscarriage.

By that afternoon I had noticed the pain was primarily on my right side. Lifting my right leg was painful, making it difficult to drive or to walk, and something didn't seem right. I was expected at work the next day but called in sick and went to see Dr Trang instead. We had already started trying for a baby and I was concerned that a night of crazy vomiting might have done some damage to my insides.

Dr Trang felt my stomach and said she thought it could be my appendix causing the pain. She tested my urine sample and found there was blood in my urine which meant an infection. She wrote a referral for the hospital and sent me straight to the emergency department for scans to get some answers.

## 37

the rupture

Jonathan met me at the hospital and we sat together in the emergency waiting room. It was so nice to have him there beside me. He had called the office and his amazing boss told him to stay with me and not to worry about coming in. I was so grateful for her kindness and understanding. I felt like we had been through so much, and every time I needed him throughout this season, she always told him to put his family first. I won't ever forget what that meant to me.

The triage nurse called me in and out a few times for assessments and a blood test before I was finally given a bed. When the doctor came in to see me with the results from my blood test he looked a little concerned. He said that my white blood count was up and the pain that I described was textbook appendicitis. He said the blood results also showed that I was about three weeks pregnant.

My heart sank. Appendicitis and pregnant. Like my body didn't have enough problems holding on to a baby. What would this mean? The doctor said that he thought it was appendicitis but because I was pregnant it could also be an ectopic pregnancy. They did a quick ultrasound but it was way too early to see anything baby-related.

I was then assessed by the surgical team who were quite certain it was my appendix and put me down on the list for surgery that evening. The doctor warned me that the infection in my body would make it hard for the baby to survive, let alone the risk from the surgery to remove my appendix.

Jonathan had been out moving the car while I was being assessed. When he returned I told him the news. It was the first time I had told him I was pregnant and a look of dread rather than joy came over him. We both had the same look. We had prayed so much for an end to our pain. We were trying so hard to live in faith when it came to growing our family. What did this timing mean?

I had a meeting with the surgeon. She told me that there was a very high risk of miscarriage, but they had no choice but to operate. In the 24 hours between arriving at the hospital and going into surgery, I'd say I was told that same line more than 20 times. Doctors, nurses and surgeons all held my hand and looked deep into my eyes.

They told me it was more than likely that this baby wasn't here to stay. But I knew that my child ultimately wasn't in their hands. He or she was in God's hands. I knew in my heart that if this baby was meant to be here then God would make a way. *"With man this is impossible, but with God all things are possible"* (Matthew 19:26).

When we started trying for the third time I knew that being pregnant after two miscarriages wasn't going to be easy. I wasn't sure how fearful I would be, but I knew that God wouldn't want me to be full of fear or anxiety while pregnant. It made me think. If this baby did survive both the infection and the surgery, would this be my sign from God that this child was here to stay? If our baby made it through this, then maybe I could trust that he or she would get through anything.

Could this be the baby that beats the odds? Was this my little miracle, my warrior child?

I spent that night praying as I waited for my surgery. Every now and then the surgeon would come in and update me on how much longer I'd have to wait. Her eyes were growing more and more weary each time she came in. It got to about midnight and I started to pray for refreshing for the surgeons who would obviously be getting tired.

About half an hour later she came back and told me that my turn was still a good four hours away and she thought it would be best to wait until tomorrow morning when the team was fresh. I was in pain, but it wasn't excruciating. I tried to get some sleep.

Thankfully I was first on the list the next morning. A team of fresh surgeons, doctors and nurses lined the hallway for a meeting to start their shift. As I was wheeled in past them all I knew that my prayers had been answered and I was in good hands.

I was pulled into a room where the anaesthetist began to prep me. I told her I was pregnant and so she went to check my chart and came back with a very concerned look on her face. She held my hand. "I need to tell you something," she said. I saw a look in her eyes that I had seen so many times before. "I just checked your blood results and your HCG levels have dropped considerably. It appears you've already lost your baby."

My heart sank. But only for a second. How could this be? I still felt in my heart that everything was ok. In fact I felt quite confident that she was wrong. But who was I to argue? Then I heard a voice in my head say "You've only had one blood test". My heart lifted. I asked the doctor how she knew my levels had dropped because I had only had one blood test since arriving at the hospital. She looked very confused and asked "Are you sure?" I nodded my head and she went off to check again.

As it turned out the surgeon had asked Dr Trang to send over all of my records, and the anaesthetist was looking at the blood test results from my last miscarriage. She was very apologetic but I told her it was ok. I felt so calm. I had spent the past 24 hours praying and had a whole church praying for me and my baby. I knew God would have His way and at that moment I was in a place of peace. I was able to hand everything over to Him. I really had no choice.

I was taken into theatre. I remember praying as I was put to sleep just like I did for Preston's birth. The surgeon said that when they finally took a look inside things were a mess. My appendix had already ruptured and caused a lot of damage. Aside from the removal of my appendix they also had to take out part of my bowel, did some heavy cleaning around my uterus and removed some adhesions from around my stomach.

The surgeon who came to see me after the surgery told me that it was pretty bad inside and they almost had to cut me right open. Thankfully they managed to do everything using only keyhole surgery. Another prayer answered. Who knows what harm major surgery could have done to our baby. I could only imagine the difference between this well-rested surgical team that morning, and the tired eyes I saw the night before. God was looking after me.

## 38

the church that prayed

I looked up at the ceiling from my hospital bed, unable to move without sharp pains shooting up through my body.

Aside from the general pain that came from removing body parts, there was also the discomfort that came from the keyhole method. My body was filled with gas during the surgery so they could find their way around. It took a few days for the gas to start to leave my body. This made it incredibly painful to sit, stand or move around. Every time I sat up I got sharp pains shooting up into my shoulder. I also found it very hard to breath, unless I was laying down.

I had two drainage tubes coming out of my stomach with a bag attached to each. I struggled to sit up, and couldn't stand on my own. The first time I attempted to walk to the bathroom I needed a wheelchair to get back to my bed. I couldn't breathe and it was so painful.

My friend Elizabeth sent me a message, which was a quote by author Mark Anthony. It said *"And one day she discovered that she was fierce, and strong, and full of fire, and that not even she could hold herself back, because her passion burned brighter than her fears."*

I read it and tears began running down the side of my face. It was so hard to stay positive and so hard to look past the present pain that I was in. But I knew that I could do it. I knew that one day, maybe a year from now, I would look back on this quote and smile again. Hopefully with a beautiful little baby in my arms.

I was so surprised by the amount of pain I was in. I had a c-section with Preston three years before and the recovery back then was much easier than it was this time around.

I made the decision that I would only take paracetamol for the pain, as I didn't want to take anything that could harm my baby. Morphene and Endone were offered many times but I just couldn't do it. This child had come so far and through so much. I didn't want to risk anything that could cause harm or damage.

Jonathan was sending regular updates to our pastor who sent out prayer requests to the entire church. We love our church so much. It had become our second home and the members were our family. I could feel their prayers working. Even through the toughest times when I struggled to get out of bed, I knew that they were lifting me in prayer. I had never been in so much pain, felt so unwell or been unable to move like that, but I still had hope and trusted in God that each day things would get better. They did.

I listened to a lot of worship music in hospital. Most of the day I had it playing through my headphones. At night it was the only way I could get to sleep. I could feel it bringing peace to my soul. I felt like the music stopped me from becoming fearful about what was ahead.

Our friends from church were sending through worship songs, videos, bible verses and uplifting prayers every day. My beautiful friend Angela messaged me to say that her family had taken communion for me and my baby, and pleaded the blood of Christ over us. This gave me so much peace. Our baby was covered with its own divine protection. Our church friends were dropping food to our house and offered to help with cleaning or babysitting, whatever we needed. They were amazing.

Slowly but surely, I was able to breath again. I managed walking a little better each day, and after a week of eating absolutely nothing, I was able to take in some food. Every morning the nurse would take some blood to check on my hormone levels and see how the baby was doing. Then, each day the doctor would let me know that the HCG levels had risen and that everything was ok for now.

I tried to stay positive. I'm not the type of person to ever wish a day away, but I wanted to fast forward to a time when I was in the clear and I could feel my baby growing inside me. Until then I had no choice but to focus on my recovery and trust in God that everything would be ok. I knew our church was praying for my heart, just as much as they prayed for my physical recovery and our baby. There's no way my heart would have survived that time in hospital without it.

# 39

## mummy's at work

I picked up my phone to call him, but instantly felt the tears form in the back of my throat. I put my phone down and cried, wiping the tears from my face with the front of my hospital gown. I had never been away from Preston for so long and I longed to hear his voice.

We were so blessed to have my mum in town the day I was admitted. She took some extra time off work and stayed at our house to look after Preston while Jonathan came to and from the hospital. We decided that we didn't want Preston to see me so unwell. We knew how much it would upset him and we didn't want him to worry about me. For the first few days we told him I was at work. I wasn't able to video call him because he would be able to tell that I wasn't ok. They sent me photos and videos of him playing and I sent him messages and letters in the mail.

One night Jonathan sent me a sound clip of his conversation with Preston as he put him to sleep. I've typed it up word for word because it's just so beautiful and shows the love and compassion in his heart.

Jonathan: What are you doing?

Preston: I'm just praying

Jonathan: What are you praying? Do you want to pray together?

Preston: It's for baby.

Jonathan: Are you praying for the baby? Aww that's nice.

Preston: And I'm praying for you and Pastor Paul.

Jonathan: That's nice, what about mummy?

Preston: Yes Jesus, look after mummy and ma ma Julz (my mum).

Jonathan: Amen

Preston: Amen

The sound of my two-year old praying got me through the next few days in that hospital bed. It was so hard to be away from him.

The recovery was taking longer than I expected. I was praying for the day that I could stand up straight and walk around without being out of breath or in pain. I followed the doctor's orders and each day walked a little further and spent more and more time out of bed sitting in my chair. Even though my mind was preoccupied with my recovery, and I was so determined to get better, I still thought of my little Preston every minute. I wondered what he was doing and I worried what he was really thinking about me being away.

Mum and Jonathan kept telling me that he was happy and easily distracted, but to me I could see a different look in his eyes in the photos they sent me. On day five they sent me a video of Preston opening a letter that I had sent him. It made me worry even more. He was obviously worried about his mum and scared. I could tell he was confused about why I had been gone for so long. I needed to see him, to show him that I was ok. I got up out of that bed and for the first time I took off my hospital gown and put on some real clothes. I practiced walking up and down the hallway until I knew I was strong enough to do it when Preston came to visit.

I knew it would be a shock to him when he came to the hospital, but my heart ached for him and I wanted him to know that everything would be ok. I asked Jonathan to bring him in the next day. We met in the hallway. It certainly was't the run and jump Hallmark moment you'd see in the movies. Preston hid behind his dad's leg and his beautiful big eyes peeked out at me. First he looked at me, then at the cannula in my hand, then up and down the hallway. I could tell he was scared and we needed to take things slowly. Preston looked at me again. I sat on the ground and he slowly came forward and gave me a hug. It had only been five days but it felt like five years. I wondered how long it would have taken for him to forget about me if the worst had happened. But then I felt my heart ache more than I could bear, and I made myself stop thinking that way.

We sat for a while and Jonathan tried to prompt Preston to tell me about his day and all of his new "surprises", but our little boy was so quiet. I held back the tears and kept a big smile on my face. Inside my heart was aching. I didn't want him to be scared, and I hoped that our bond would be restored quickly. After he seemed a bit more comfortable Jonathan said he had to go and get something from the car and left us alone. I was a little scared that he wouldn't want to stay with me, but he did.

We sat and looked at the helipad outside and made small talk. I let him pretend to fill his Percy toy up with 'fuel' from my cannula and before I knew it he had his arms wrapped around my neck hugging me from the back. When Jono returned he managed to get a photo of that moment. It's one I won't ever forget. When it was time for them to leave I showed Preston where I would be sleeping, and said that Dr Trang needed me to stay a little bit longer while she fixed my belly. He asked if he could come back tomorrow to pick me up?

The next day he did just that. I was discharged from hospital.

*40*

---

# rings of fire

I followed the doctor's orders and rested at home. Our church friends continued to drop in meals for us, and my mum stayed to help look after Preston while I recovered.

My beautiful friend's Hazel and Michelle from work turned up on my door step with a big bunch of flowers. We worked at the local council for the mayor and general manager, and they said everyone was so worried about me. They had all been so supportive through our miscarriages and allowed me to take all the time I needed to grieve our babies. As I recovered from my appendix rupture they were just as lovely in giving me time to rest. Hazel and Michelle had come to the hospital the day after my surgery and saw me at my worst. I think they were surprised to see me out of bed answering the door a week later. It was nice to spend time with them. When it was time to leave they passed on strict orders not to look at any work emails, or even think about work until I had fully recovered. I was so grateful for this.

As each day got a little easier, my mind refocussed on our baby. I was only home a couple of days when some cramping started. I was so exhausted and in pain, and I wondered if this was it? Had my body been through too much to hold on to this sweet little one? Were the doctors right? Was this baby's time up? I hoped that because the baby had survived this far that everything would be ok. I prayed and prayed and hoped for the best. The cramping lasted about 12 hours and by the next morning it stopped. By this stage I was almost five weeks pregnant and we still had to wait three more weeks for an ultrasound to see if everything was ok.

While I was in hospital my friend Rebecca was praying for me and said that God had given her a vision of me standing, holding a full-term baby with chubby cheeks. She said there were rings of fire surrounding me and the baby, like God was showing her how much fire He had been through for this child. When I first heard this, tears flooded down my face. A spiritual battle had been fought and won for me. After all I had been through in the physical, God had fought for me behind the scenes in the spiritual, and my chubby-cheeked baby would be ok.

I hung on so tightly to her vision for the next few months. Every time fear or doubt came over me I would pray and thank God for all He had done for me and this baby. As hard as it was I tried to stay in that hopeful place, believing and trusting that this baby had already come so far and was here to stay.

I was so grateful for every passing week. I thanked God for every day of morning sickness, and all of the other joyful pregnancy symptoms that came. I was determined to thank Him for this baby, all the days of my life.

## 41

the first ultrasound

It was a long wait but we finally made it to eight weeks and our first chance to see our baby. As Jonathan drove to the imaging centre we prayed that whatever the results were, God would be in that room with us, and we trusted Him to get us through it. I was really nervous but I had a good feeling about this one. I had not reached this far in my pregnancies with Gabriel or Raphie, and I felt so happy to have an opportunity to see my baby on the screen.

We were called in for our turn and I gave the nurse a brief rundown of what we had been through. I told her about the operation and the high chance of miscarriage so that she was prepared for whatever she might find.

As the transducer rolled over my stomach Jonathan and I stared intently at the screen. My heart was in my throat again. I held my breath. Then after a few seconds, there it was. A tiny, fast-paced heartbeat racing on the screen. The sweetest sound I've ever heard. We both looked at each other and tears welled in our eyes. The nurse measured the baby and took a few images. She said we had a perfectly healthy baby with a strong heart beat on our hands. I can't begin to explain the relief. I felt my heart in my throat as tears ran down the side of my face.

We walked outside and I burst into tears. Jonathan stopped on the footpath and put his arms around me. Everything was going to be ok. Our baby had made it, through the infection and the surgery our baby had held on. Those words "perfectly healthy baby with a strong heartbeat" bounced around in my head. I sent this out via text message to all of our friends and family waiting on the news.

When we sat in the car Jonathan said that he kept thinking about what could have been if Gabriel was still inside me when my appendix ruptured. I would have been seven months pregnant and an appendix rupture like mine in the third trimester could have been so much more dangerous for our baby. He said that maybe God had saved us from something much more heartbreaking, who knows?

Who knows how long it could have taken us to move forward if we lost a baby that way. We had no idea why things happened the way they did, but we were so grateful for that little heartbeat. That heartbeat brought us peace, it brought us joy and it brought us hope for the future. If God could get our baby through the first tumultuous weeks of his life, then surely the next 32 would be a breeze.

# 42

---

## fear

I felt that the Lord wanted me to pick up my laptop today, even though I really don't want to be doing it. It's been almost five weeks since my surgery and ten days since my ultrasound. Ten days since the total joy of seeing our little baby's heart beat on that screen.

I'm now nine weeks pregnant and suffering with bad pain in my lower abdomen. It feels like cramping, much like my miscarriages did, but a little different with short sharp pains occurring every few seconds. To say I'm worried would be an understatement.

I've prayed. I've told God I trust Him and I'm hoping that this will pass. It's so hard not to be consumed by fear. Especially after everything that's happened. I'm not sure what else I can do. My mind starts to race and I begin to think of all the appointments I'll need to cancel, all the friends I need to tell. Am I going to have to choose a name for another unborn baby? No. Stop.

Don't give in to those thoughts Michelle. Don't let the fear take hold. It might be different this time. It has to be different this time. What if things don't work out? Then this will be the last time. I can't do this again.

As my mind is spiralling into all the places that it's not meant to go, I begin to worry about what's physically going to happen if this is a miscarriage. Gabriel was seven weeks and Raphie was only five weeks old. This baby is nine weeks. Is that why the pain is much more intense? Am I going to see something different if this baby passes?

I'm terrified to go to the bathroom. I don't even want to stand up because if I see or feel any blood my heart will break. I don't know what that heartbreak is going to look like this time, but I fear it won't be pretty. Jonathan is at work. If only I could hold my bladder until he got home. I'm scared of what my reaction might be if I see blood in the toilet. Whatever my reaction, I don't want Preston to see it.

In between all the panic and fear, every now and then, the pain stops and I think, wait, maybe it's just surgery pains. Maybe the baby is ok. I try to remember the last time I felt morning sickness. I know I felt it yesterday but not as strong as usual. I close my eyes to pray the biggest prayer of my life, but "Lord please" were the only two words I could manage.

I decided to put on some worship music. "*Here's my heart*" by David Crowder came over the speaker. I was in the kitchen attempting to empty the dishwasher and without warning began to sob uncontrollably. I quickly stuck my head in the cupboard to put some bowls away and burst into tears. "Please God. I can't. I can't do this again. Please."

I couldn't breathe. I couldn't take my head out of the cupboard. I couldn't bear for Preston to see me like this again. I began to think about the future. I knew my heart couldn't do this again. So that would be it. Preston wouldn't have a sibling. Maybe we could adopt. My mind was racing faster than my heart. Where was the promise? Where was the rejoicing? How could this be, after all we had been through? Lord, speak to me.

My heart felt so heavy. I slowed my breathing, turned the music down and I could hear Him. "Trust me", he whispered. I felt numb. All I could feel was the pain in my uterus. I wanted to trust Him. I remembered back to Gabriel, when "Trust me" meant trust me in the good and the bad, trust me that I will hold your heart together through it all. Was this the same trust me? Or was He saying trust me that everything will be ok?

Things weren't looking good. I messaged my friend Natalie and asked her to pray. She sent me this verse:

"Peace I leave with you; my peace I give you. I do not give to you as the world gives. Do not let your hearts be troubled and do not be afraid."

Peace, how I longed to feel that peace in my heart again. How long would I have to wait for it?

Then I remembered Psalm 130:5. "I wait for the Lord my soul waits, and in His word I hope."

By the time Jonathan got home from work I was in so much pain and struggling to get Preston to sleep in his room. He came in and took over so I could lay down. I was so glad he was home. Once Preston was asleep Jonathan came to sit with me and I burst into tears again.

"I can't do this again," I cried. "I can't. I just can't."

We didn't speak, I just cried and cried. There were no words left. I was so tired, I was done. It felt like all hope was lost. I didn't want to be sad anymore. I didn't want to keep trying over and over knowing it would end in heartache. I didn't want to think past tomorrow and I spent all night terrified to go to the bathroom.

## 43

limbo

We were officially in limbo and there was nothing we could do but wait and hope for a miracle. I spent that night praying every time I went to the bathroom. Looking down at that toilet paper in total fear and anguish. I would hold my breath until I could see there was no blood, then I would breathe again.

I woke up the next morning and I didn't feel sick. The pain had subsided to an uncomfortable feeling but my morning sickness had gone. It was the first time in my life I actually wanted to feel sick but didn't. I didn't know what this meant. Had I miscarried without any bleeding? Would I need a procedure to remove the baby? What happened if you lost your baby at nine weeks? How do they get it out? What would my baby look like if they removed him or her?

I messaged a few friends some panicked questions about the pain and the morning sickness stopping. I wanted to see if they had experienced anything similar. Some had days without being sick at all. Others said they felt pain as their uterus stretched. But nobody could ease my fears. That was probably the longest day of my life. We had a swimming lesson that morning. I wasn't sure if we should go. Half an hour poolside with my own thoughts could be dangerous.

One of the other mums at swimming knew that I was pregnant. She asked how I was feeling. I lied and told her I was ok. Here I was faking it again. It was spring time so she excitedly pointed out all the other mums at the pool with big pregnant bellies. I listened as she explained that she was too old to have any more children, but she was thinking about adopting one so her two-year-old daughter could have a sibling.

Was that my problem? Was I too old to have another baby? I was almost 34. I knew lots of mums who had babies at this age. I sat and listened and joined in the baby talk. I had become pretty good at faking it. I watched Preston swim the best he's ever swum and thought maybe life wouldn't be so bad with one kid. I had already made sure he had lots of friends around him. He was close to his cousins. There was no lack of love or fun in his life.

Then I heard a voice in my head say "stop!" I realised I was giving up. I was trying to make a life in my head that was ok without my baby, and that wasn't trusting in God. I thought back to that ultrasound. That beautiful heartbeat on the screen. I made a decision that I needed to fight the good fight. I needed to snap out of it. So far there was no bleeding and God had told me to trust Him. There was still hope. With God there is always hope. I couldn't give up. I refused to give up.

I got home and turned my worship music on and prayed. I had no control over this situation but I had to trust the One who did. I had to believe that this baby had made it through the infection and the rupture and the surgery for a reason. I had to believe that this baby was here to stay. I had to trust and hold on to that promise. God told me we would rejoice and I believed with my whole heart that we would be rejoicing over this child. I wanted so desperately for everything to be ok and I needed to start believing that it would be.

There were four weeks until my next ultrasound. Such a long time to wait for answers. I was so sure that the pain I felt meant we were losing our baby. Looking back I wish I could have been more faithful. I wish I could have rested in His peace and hope, rather than panicking.

I know the Lord was with me in my distress, trying so hard to get through to me and ease my fears. But sometimes, when you're in the fire, it can be so hard to stay positive. I found it really difficult. I felt that I had come so far but then felt so bad that I couldn't totally let go and trust God that everything was ok. I told my friend Penny how bad I felt to be so full of fear. She said "God has big shoulders Mish, He knows your heart and He feels everything that you do." She was right. If I could keep being honest with God about how I was feeling, then He would keep giving me all that I needed to get through this.

A few days later, the pain slowly subsided and my morning sickness returned. I felt pregnant again. I had to keep my mind from wandering into dark places. I knew I had to keep my eyes on Jesus and keep giving thanks for this child.

## 44

# an anchor for the soul

The bible says that hope is an anchor for the soul. That verse has never meant more to me than now.

Sometimes when we are on a journey like this, it can feel like hope is all we have. When doctors and specialists aren't able to give us any answers then sometimes it can be hard to find a safe place to put your hope and your heart's most precious desires. Before I found Christ, I think the word hope had a very different meaning to what it means to me today.

Before, all I could really do was just hope for the best in all things. My hope wasn't in God, which means at different times throughout my life it was in my own hands, and the hands of other people. When my hope wasn't in God then the things I hoped for relied heavily on others and on myself, which isn't always easy, and isn't always safe.

There have been times when our situation seemed hopeless and God didn't answer our prayers, making it even harder to persevere and to hold on to that hope in our hearts. When I became a mum I'd love to say that my heart became stronger, but in actual fact I feel like my heart became more fragile. It certainly was more full of love, but at the same time there's the worry, the heartache, the anxiety and that raw emotion that comes with being a parent. You love your child so much and want the best for them so badly, that your heart can literally ache.

I think it's really only our hope and trust in God that can strengthen our hearts to survive parenthood and all the heartache, challenges and fears we face. Today, now that I know Jesus, I feel like the word hope carries a lot more weight. With God, hope is much more significant. My hope is in Him no matter what I'm going through. I know where my hope lies and I know that I can trust Him with all my hopes and dreams.

When it comes to our desires sometimes the things we hope for don't always go to plan and that's when hope can feel quite heavy in our hearts. When there's pain, suffering and heartache, sometimes it's hard to have hope, but then at the same time hope can literally be all we have. That's when it becomes important that we persevere in hope and that we don't give up.

Romans 5:2-7 says that *"suffering produces perseverance; perseverance, character and character, hope. And hope does not put us to shame, because God's love has been poured out into our hearts through the Holy Spirit who has been given to us."*

God can use our suffering to build our character and create a brand new hope in us. As a mum I feel like my perseverance and character are growing and developing each day. When we lost Gabriel and Raphie I felt like my heart and soul were smashed to pieces and I needed that anchor. I needed that hope.

By persevering in hope, our character is developed. We become stronger and more resilient. We learn to draw on God's strength and in turn we can hand over our worries about the future and hold on to that hope that things will turn out for good, that joy will come after the storm.

Some days I look at myself now, compared to before I met Jonathan, before I knew the Lord, before my journey through miscarriage and I don't recognise who I see. Looking back now, I can see how far I have come, and how much hope I have, because of my relationship with Jesus.

I am so grateful that my hope is safe in His hands. I am so in awe of His goodness and His grace. I am so grateful for that anchor.

# 45

## 12 weeks

We finally made it past 12 weeks and the anxiety about miscarriage began to subside. I had made it much further than the past two pregnancies and was still feeling sick and pregnant. My belly was growing and people were starting to notice and get excited for us. I was just waiting on my next scan to make sure everything was ok.

At 12 weeks, we were booked in for an ultrasound. It was a Friday morning and it was raining. Initially we wanted to take Preston with us, but we decided against it. The pains I had a few weeks ago were fresh in my mind and if something was wrong with our baby I didn't want Preston there to see it.

We packed him in the car with Grandma Julz and sent them off to playgroup, or the "sandpit school" as he called it. It was a local playgroup with a huge sandpit full of trucks, diggers and all the things Preston loved to play with. I knew he would be safe and have a great morning and I hoped we would too.

Jonathan came with me. He was flying to Melbourne for work that morning but had half an hour to spend with us before he left. I was so grateful for that. Half an hour would give us time to hear the heartbeat and hopefully see our baby move around the screen. As soon as the doppler touched my stomach an image of the most beautiful, perfectly-formed baby, came up on the screen. We watched in awe as our baby moved around, even lifting its hand up to give us what looked like a wave. It was so perfect. I closed my eyes and thought "What a miracle". In that moment I truly felt that everything was going to be ok.

The nurse took all the measurements and asked me a series of questions. She printed out a few of the photos for me to take home. She said the rest would be available with the report after the blood test results came in. I had seen my baby and had the most beautiful photos to take home so I wasn't concerned about the rest. I went to have my blood test and headed home.

The next day we decided it was time to tell the world, or I should say tell "our world" about our baby. I remember with Preston I couldn't wait to get on social media and tell everyone our exciting news. I think it was 12 weeks exactly when we announced our little bundle was on its way. This time was different though. A lot of people already knew about our baby because of my appendix and our urgent need for prayer support. There were others however who didn't know because we had been so afraid something might go wrong.

We decided to keep the positive vibes going and share our news on social media. We took a cute photo of Preston sitting on our lounge holding the ultrasound up in the air like a proud big brother. The post read "How blessed you are already little one to call this guy your big brother. Baby Ng due April 2018."

My cousin Karen who I had kept up to date with everything we had been through was keeping our pregnancy a secret. She messaged me to say her daughter Emily just saw the post and was "joyously shouting out the beautiful news". She then told me that she had planted two olive trees in her garden for Gabriel and Raphie. She said she chose olives because of our Mediterranean heritage and because the olive branch is a symbol of peace. As I read her message my heart ached and my eyes filled with tears. Such a beautiful idea to remember my babies and I hoped a sign of what was to come. I couldn't wait to hold my precious baby in my arms and finally feel some peace.

# charlotte's web

It was Thursday afternoon, almost a week after my ultrasound. Preston and I were sitting on the lounge watching *Charlotte's Web* together. The weather was gloomy outside and someone in our street had put fertiliser on their lawn. My pregnant nose couldn't handle the smell so we closed all the windows and sat on the lounge with our pillows.

Preston had just stopped his day naps, so by this time of day we were both exhausted and ready to crash. It was way too late in the afternoon for him to sleep though. I couldn't risk him being awake half the night as a result.

The movie had just started when my phone rang. I looked at the screen and saw it was my doctor calling. I was a bit confused and headed into our kitchen to answer. It was Dr Has, he said he was keeping an eye on Dr Trang's patients while she was away, and he needed to talk to me about my results. My brain was a bit foggy and I couldn't think what results he was talking about.

I wasn't expecting a call or waiting on any results. "I'm sorry, which results?" I asked him. He told me the results from the ultrasound and blood tests, and asked me to come and see him on Monday to discuss them. He then asked if I was seeing an obstetrician? I said no. I was due to have my first appointment with my midwife next week and didn't plan on seeing an obstetrician. He asked me if I could ring and book an appointment with an obstetrician and then come in on Monday to get the referral and have a chat.

I was still confused. I told him that Monday was a few days away and asked if I needed to be worried? He asked if Dr Trang had explained what the ultrasound would be testing for? I told him she mentioned Down Syndrome but I really only had the ultrasound because I had two miscarriages this year. I just wanted to check the baby was still growing.

He said the results took into consideration certain measurements of the baby and the blood results to determine the risk factor for Down Syndrome. He didn't go into too much detail on the phone but said there was further testing that could be done to determine more accurately if our baby had Down Syndrome. He said there were risks involved in this testing that he would explain to me on Monday.

I told him that if our baby had Down Syndrome we wouldn't be terminating the pregnancy so any tests that were a risk to our baby wouldn't be considered. He said that was one of the things he was going to ask me when I came in. He said if I wanted to book the obstetrician to make sure I got an appointment, then after Monday when I have all the information I can cancel the appointment if I needed to.

I hung up the phone shocked, confused and lost for words. I wanted to cry but I didn't know exactly why. Perhaps it was the shock. I wanted to pray but I didn't know what to say. I didn't want to seem ungrateful for this baby because I wasn't. I still loved him or her with all my heart. Ultimately I didn't care if our baby had Down Syndrome or not. During my time as a journalist I had met so many beautiful children and adults who had the syndrome and they were all the sweetest, most amazing people.

I don't think Down Syndrome was the issue. Perhaps the shock came because I wasn't expecting any results from that scan at all. I had seen the baby's heartbeat and it was measuring at the right size. I had totally forgotten that there were more results coming. The phone call from Dr Has seemed totally out of the blue. For him to want a serious conversation with me in person had me in shock. I just needed some time to process it.

I messaged my friend Heather and told her I felt lost. She told me the devil was trying to distract me from the miracle, and came over straight away to pray with me. I was careful not to pray for a child without Down Syndrome. I didn't want to pray against God's will and I certainly didn't want to speak out that I didn't want a baby with Down Syndrome. We prayed for a healthy baby and thanked God for the miracle that this baby was to us. I wanted whatever baby God was going to give me. Heather and her husband David went into battle for us. They marked the date in their calendar and prayed together every day for 40 days for our baby. I won't ever forget how much this meant to me.

I knew in my heart that no matter what the results, everything would be ok. But I was being attacked by fear. My mind raced thinking about the future. How different our lives might be. What this would mean for Preston? Would our children need to go to different schools? Would we need to build a granny flat out the back to make sure that our child could live independently one day, and still have us there for support? What would I need to do to

149

ensure this baby had the best life and opportunities possible despite the circumstances?

Jonathan and I lifted our game and began praying together every night for our children. We prayed scripture verses over them both, and I put an ultrasound photo on the wall in our wardrobe with scripture verses written around it. We wanted to be thankful for our baby no matter what and we wanted God's will to be done. Over the next few days God gave us such peace in our hearts about this child. It became obvious that God had orchestrated my appointment with the doctor to be four days after that phone call. It gave us both time to grow and stretch in our faith.

By Sunday afternoon I felt nothing but love and excitement again for our baby. The fear was gone and there was a total peace that everything was as it should be. We knew that no matter what happened God would give us what we needed for this baby. To us a healthy baby included a baby with Down Syndrome. We had wanted and prayed for this child and God had already answered our prayers.

## 47

# high risk

The next morning I dropped in to the imaging centre to pick up my scan results. Dr Has had already told me some information on the phone but I was still interested to read the results myself. I opened the oversized envelope and my eyes were immediately drawn to dark bold text in capital letters at the bottom of the page – HIGH RISK DOWN SYNDROME.

My heart skipped a beat. Seeing it in writing made things a little more real and a little less clear. My mind felt like it was in a fog. I didn't realise that there were different levels of risk. I wondered what "high" risk actually meant. Did this mean that it was probable or did it just mean that compared to others my risk factors were higher? I skimmed the pages of the report eagerly looking for more answers. Numbers, I needed numbers. Then I read, ratio: 1/71.

Compared to other medical conditions which could have a one in a thousand, or one in a million chance, this was quite high. But mathematically a one in seventy one chance didn't seem so bad. I messaged my brother Michael; who was always much better at maths than I was. He said that it was less than two percent and he told me I should stay positive, because everything would be ok. I was tempted to Google but that has never helped me in the past. I prayed and handed it to God. Something it seemed I would need to do over and over again for the rest of this pregnancy. As I drove to playgroup that morning, the words HIGH RISK rolled around in my brain, like two marbles on a wooden floor, making so much noise I could barely hear anything else.

Until God spoke.

"Stop," he said. "Be still".

I stopped to listen and all of a sudden several parts of bible verses began flooding my mind again:

*"Fearfully and wonderfully made"*

*"In his image"*

*"You knit me together in my mothers womb"*

*"I know the plans I have for you, plans of hope and a future"*

*"Not by strength or by might but by my spirit."*

God's plans for this baby had already been decided. No amount of fear or worrying could change that. The devil could try with all his might to distract me from the miracle and take away my joy, but I was determined not to let him. It didn't matter if my baby had Down syndrome, my baby is still perfect. My baby is still a gift from the Lord. My baby is still meant to be here.

A spiritual battle was raging and I had to fight. I remembered what Rebecca had told me about the rings of fire. I thought about what God had already been through for this child, and for me and Jonathan. I had to stay in a place of hope and joy and thanksgiving. I knew that God would never give up on me, so I had to make sure I wasn't giving up on Him.

*48*

---

# only human

Despite my trust in God, which was a continual journey, I was only human. I trusted God to look after my baby but I also had a desire for answers. It was Monday morning and I was sitting in the waiting room at the doctor's surgery. I wondered what Dr Has would have to say. I had a list of questions for him and the scan results in my hand. I guess I just wanted facts from him and was hoping he would support my decision to forgo any further testing. Jonathan and I had made the decision that this baby's fate was better left in God's hands and we didn't need to know any more than that. On a spiritual level this seemed the right thing to do. The human side of me wanted more information.

Dr Has went through my options. These included an amniocentesis which involved using a thin needle to withdraw a small amount of fluid from the sac surrounding the baby. There was a risk of miscarriage associated with this test, so obviously our answer was no. We were also offered a non-invasive blood test called the Harmony Test, which was around $400 and would be 99% accurate to screen for Down Syndrome. Most people would opt for this test, but we felt like it wouldn't make much difference to us. While part of me wanted to know, another part didn't need to.

Dr Has accepted our decision not to progress with further testing because no matter what the outcome, we wouldn't be terminating the pregnancy. I loved how supportive he was and was grateful that he respected our decision. He wanted me to see an obstetrician regardless just to have that extra support. I took the referral home but never used it. If we were going to do anything it would be the Harmony Test but there was something stopping me from going down that path. I can definitely see why people would do it, to be more prepared, but we didn't feel our preparation for this baby would be any different whether he or she had Down Syndrome or not. All we wanted to do was be excited and love this baby and be thankful for the miracle growing inside me. So that's exactly what we did.

I had a phone call with the genetic counsellors from the hospital and told them why we didn't want to do any further testing. This baby was a miracle and a blessing and it didn't matter what the results. They wrote a letter to my midwife and from then on, nobody mentioned further testing to us. We were able to enjoy the pregnancy for what it was, a beautiful baby to complete our beautiful family.

## 49

# feel the joy

We made it to 19 weeks and up until now there had been more worry and fear around this pregnancy than we'd like to admit. Even as the morning sickness subsided that became a worry that something was wrong, when usually it would be a time of great relief. I thought back to my first pregnancy with Preston and how joyful that was.

I spent a lot of my first pregnancy working away from home in Canberra and I remember returning at the end of each week to see the look on Jonathan's face when my belly had grown bigger. Things back then were so exciting and I never for a second worried that something could go wrong.

This pregnancy was different. It was a constant battle to hold on to my peace. I had to remind myself every day to trust in God, and to hand this baby over to Him every time I felt the fear creeping in. It's so hard to totally let go when your heart's desire is so great and in reach.

On the way to our 19 week scan I felt excited and nervous at the same time. As we drove the short drive to the imaging centre, I asked Jonathan how he would feel if we found out the gender of our baby.

"Everything has been so stressful and I just want to feel some joy," I said to him. He held my hand and smiled. "Let's do it babe!" he said.

I knew that whether our baby was a boy or a girl I would be so excited and it would give me something to focus on rather than keeping him or her alive. We'd be able to choose a name and get the nursery ready. Knowing the gender would allow me to fall even more in love with this baby and form a deeper connection to the little life inside me. I knew this would be a good thing, even if the worst was to happen. I wanted a strong connection to this baby so badly, because I felt my time was cut so short with Gabriel and Raphie.

We agreed not to tell anyone that we knew the gender of our baby. We wanted to surprise our family and friends when the time came. I immediately thought of the few people I had trouble keeping secrets from and wondered how long I could keep it from them. The nurse took all the images she needed, then gave us a guided tour of my uterus. She was just about to wrap things up when I asked her if she could tell what the gender was. She moved the doppler around and said "are you sure you want to know?" I looked at Jonathan, we smiled at each other and he said "yes".

She smiled and pointed to the screen "well this one is pretty obvious" she said. "It's a boy!". I immediately felt tears of joy in my throat. My heart skipped a beat. Another beautiful boy and a best friend for Preston. I was overjoyed and I couldn't remove the grin from my face.

Finally in my mind I could piece together a future with this baby and it felt so real. From that moment on, I wasn't worried about miscarriage or Down Syndrome. I began to feel the joy in my heart and I truly believed that nothing could take my little boy away from me.

## 50

*irreplaceable*

On Gabriel's due date I was about 15 weeks pregnant and on Raphie's due date I was 26 weeks. Preston was so curious and eager to understand everything that was going on, so I was reluctant to include him in anything to remember our babies this year. I didn't want to confuse him by talking about the babies who went to heaven, or have him worry about his little brother for the rest of the pregnancy. He had already been through enough.

A couple of friends messaged to say they were thinking of me and I spent some quiet time in prayer asking God to hug my babies and make sure they knew I hadn't forgotten them. I lit a candle for each of them and had a quiet cry on my own. In the years to come I'm sure we will remember our babies as a family. I want to think of something unique for each of them that we can do together to celebrate and to make sure we don't forget.

I'm not sure how different this year would have been if I wasn't pregnant when the due dates came around. I can only imagine the heartache and great sense of loss in knowing that you should be getting ready to give birth. Being pregnant didn't take away the pain for me, but it did remind me that this baby was meant to be here, and that he wouldn't be if my other pregnancies were successful.

Whether you're pregnant or not on your baby's due date, hold on tight to that hope that the baby who is meant to be here will be in your arms one day, and you won't be able to imagine your life any other way. The thought of not having the child who made it into your arms is just as heartbreaking as losing the ones who didn't.

To me, Gabriel and Raphie are irreplaceable. Their due dates certainly pulled on my heartstrings, but also gave me a chance to be grateful for the little life growing inside me. This baby didn't replace them. But this baby is the one who I would one day hold in my arms. This baby will be the one I couldn't imagine my life without.

# 51

## he's not moving

The final few months of my pregnancy were the longest of my life. My body struggled this time around and there was little I could do to make things better. I was exhausted and trying to keep up with Preston became harder and harder. The days were long that's for sure. Jonathan was still working the afternoon shift and I was so tired that I decided to change Preston's routine so he had a 6pm bed time. It meant waking up earlier but at least I could plonk on the lounge earlier each night once he was asleep.

This baby was super active in the womb. He was so different to Preston that I couldn't believe it. I knew this was God's way of easing any anxiety I had about my baby. Preston was delivered six weeks early due to decreased movement caused by a blood clot in my umbilical cord. If you add that to my two miscarriages, you would expect to have a pretty anxious mumma on your hands, even at this late stage in my pregnancy. I needed to feel my baby move to know that he was ok.

Our baby boy already had his own routine and I could see a pattern with his movements. Aside from feeling him move quite often throughout the day, when I sat down at night to watch television with Jonathan, the baby would move around so much that we could sit back and watch him. Each time I would look up at the clock and it would be around 9pm.

I was 36 weeks plus three days when things changed. I had to force myself to sit still a few times throughout the day and eat chocolate or an ice block to try and get him moving again. It felt like his movements had slowed considerably and I began to worry. "Surely not" the voice inside my head would say. "There's no way this could happen again". I prayed that the Lord would give me a sign if I needed to go to the hospital.

After Preston was born the doctor said that what happened was a one-time event and there was no reason it should happen again with future pregnancies. I could feel the fear creeping in again. 9pm came and there were no movements. Why was he so still? I couldn't sleep that night. Usually laying still in bed would promote a second round of movements sometime after midnight but not this time. Every time I made the decision to get out of bed and call the hospital he would move again. Surely I was being paranoid.

The next morning I dropped Preston at my mum's house and drove to see the midwife at our local hospital. She had a student nurse helping her for the day. They called me in for my appointment and I sat down, hoping the usual chit chat wouldn't last long so we could listen to the baby's heartbeat.

The first question she asked hit me like an arrow to the heart. "How are the baby's movements?" she said.

I burst into tears and shook my head.

"He's not moving".

# 52

## somersaults

The midwife took my hand and asked me to lay down on the bed. "Why didn't you call when you realised he wasn't moving?" she asked. "You of all people know it's important to call."

She put the gel on the end of the doppler and I closed my eyes and prayed or perhaps the right word is begged, "Please Lord let me hear that sweet sound, please let there be a heartbeat." As the gel hit my skin I could hear my insides sloshing around for a few seconds, then finally a heart beat. Tears ran down my face and on to the pillow. The trainee gave me a tissue and the nurse kept the doppler on my stomach for a minute or two while I listened and cried.

She told me she was going to send me to the specialised antenatal unit at another hospital to monitor the baby for a while, if anything, to put my mind at ease. I was grateful. She rushed through the rest of the check up, called the hospital to book me in and sent me over there straight away. On the way to the hospital the sun shone down on my car much like the day I drove myself to have Preston checked out when he wasn't moving. I remembered it so vividly and did exactly the same thing all the way there, I prayed.

161

I prayed for protection for the baby and thanked God for a strong heartbeat and a healthy baby. I thanked God for everything He had done so far to keep my baby safe. I thought back to those rings of fire and felt so grateful that I had Christ on my side. This baby was meant to be here and I knew he was going to grow up to do amazing things. Despite hearing the heartbeat I still hadn't felt the baby move since the previous night. It was so different to the usual acrobatics I felt happening inside me.

When I arrived at the hospital I was taken to a room full of pregnant women hooked up to machines monitoring their babies. Some looked nervous, others were on their phones looking bored. A large strap was placed around my stomach attached to a monitor where the sound of the heartbeat came through the speaker. It came through loud and strong.

The nurse told me to rest and press a button whenever I felt the baby move. I laid back and waited. I prayed for a sign from the Lord that everything was ok. It only took a few minutes before my baby got the message. All of a sudden the movements in my stomach were so intense that the sound coming from the machine sounded like a windstorm on the other end of a mobile phone. The nurse raced in and turned the volume down on my machine. We both stared at my stomach and watched as my baby poked and stretched and danced around inside me.

"He's doing somersaults in there!" the nurse said.

I smiled and placed one hand on my stomach. The somersaults were my sign from God. My baby was ok.

## 53

## my little warrior

It was Jonathan who named Preston. At first I wasn't convinced on the name but it grew on me. Then during our stay in hospital I realised it was the perfect name for our little man. This time around it was a bit different. We had just named two babies that we couldn't hold in our arms or kiss goodnight. We chose Gabriel Luca and Raphie Jay because we loved the meanings of their names and felt they suited our babies in heaven.

This little one was different again. He was a survivor. My little warrior. He had beaten the odds and was such a miracle. Every doctor and nurse who saw my scars continued to be amazed that he had survived. He was meant to be here and we needed a strong name to suit the blessing.

We decided on Theodore Louis.

Theodore means a gift from God and Louis means warrior. I knew this little boy was so strong and resilient and I knew that God must have amazing plans for him. My little warrior who had survived so much, would one day be a true warrior in God's army.

Louis is also the name of my pop who passed away the week we found out that I was pregnant. He was a warrior himself, a soldier in the Maltese Army during World War II and a prayer warrior for his family. A hero in both respects.

This was the first name we came up with and it stuck. Every now and then we discussed it and couldn't think of a better fit. Theodore Louis would soon be here to complete our family and I couldn't wait to hold my sweet baby boy in my arms.

## 54

## our hearts rejoiced

Due to the unusual circumstances of Preston's birth, this time around was ultimately my first experience of labour and child birth. I wasn't sure what to expect but spent a lot of time in prayer and studying the word to combat any fear or anxiety around giving birth. When the time came I wasn't sure if I was as ready as I should be.

From the moment those contractions started, I could feel my mind haze over, unable to focus on anything but the pain. In a nutshell, I spent 20 hours at home with painful contractions ten minutes apart. Jonathan sat up with me through the night timing my contractions. We were both exhausted and I wasn't sure how much more I could take.

After 20 hours I called the birthing unit at the hospital. They recommended staying at home until those contractions sped up. I hung up the phone and cried. I was physically and emotionally exhausted. I had no idea how much longer this would go on for, and wondered if I had it in me. I sent out an SOS message to my church small group and asked for some back up in prayer.

My friend Natalie was the first to reply, she always fills me with so much hope.

"All of heaven is backing you, you've got everything you need to do this!," she said.

"I believe you are 'strengthened with all might according to His glorious power'."

It's amazing how words that line up with the word of God can give you what you need. In my case it was some courage to go on. I'm not sure what those girls prayed but within minutes of my text my contractions sped up from ten minutes apart to five minutes and then two minutes apart. It was such a miracle. So much so that I made Jonathan call the midwife this time because I knew she wouldn't believe me that things had changed so quickly.

Jonathan put Preston to sleep and my mum came over to babysit while we went to the hospital. I had four contractions within the fifteen minute drive to get there, and then another in the hospital foyer. By the time Jonathan had parked the car and come back inside, I was already being wheeled to the birthing unit by a hospital orderly. I had another contraction as we reached the nurse's desk and was taken into our room.

The nurse checked me over and said I was 8cm dilated so it was too late for any pain medication but things were progressing nicely. For the past nine months I had a picture of what labour and childbirth would be like and how things would play out for us. I imagined that there would be pain, but in my mind there would also be an element of beauty and romance about it all. I pictured Jonathan holding my hand and looking into my eyes as I pushed our baby out, with our favourite worship song playing in the background.

Well the worship music was playing, but everything else was very different. In fact I'm not sure how much of the worship music was heard over my screaming with every push. It was intense. I prayed through every contraction and pushed as hard as I could whenever they told me to. I looked over to the small bed with lights, a heater and oxygen, ready for Theodore once he was born. My heart ached. I remembered back three years ago looking at the same bed in the corner before Preston arrived.

I'd love to say that the thought I could be holding this baby in my arms within minutes took over and the pain subsided, but it did not. Things were intense. Jonathan was a great support. He kept reminding me to breathe and stuck close by my side. At one point he reminded me that it was my beautiful friend Prue's birthday for two more hours. Prue is my oldest friend and has known me since before I was born. I was excited that my warrior baby might share a birthday with her, to me she is the ultimate warrior.

We soon got to a point where I had to get the baby out fast. He had done a poo in the womb which could be quite dangerous if he was in there any longer. I was given a episiotomy (a surgical cut made to aid a difficult delivery) and awaited the next contraction to push again.

I can remember pushing as hard as possible and the doctor telling me to keep pushing as long as the contraction was going. The contraction stopped, so I stopped. The nurse told me to lose the gas because it was distracting me from the job at hand. So I did. The next contraction came and I pushed with all my might. There were four nurses, an obstetrician, a paediatrician and a loving husband in the room all cheering me on. I can't remember what any of them were saying, but I remember the moment the baby finally came out and they lifted him straight up on to my chest.

It was done.

I caught my breath. I looked at my beautiful child and tears filled my eyes. I remembered Gabriel and Raphie, I remembered how broken I was and the dark place I was in. The past 12 months of heartache, guts and determination, pressing into the Lord, had brought me to this point. The courage to try for another baby after losing two had been worth it. He was finally here and my heart was so full. It was time to rejoice and in that special moment nothing else in this world mattered. I was laying in bed, sweat still dripping from my forehead, my cheeks rosy, my hair a tangled mess, holding my sweet, sweet baby boy in my arms.

He was perfect.

The Lord had answered our prayers and blessed us with a healthy little boy. Theodore Louis Ng was here.

Thinking back to this moment my heart aches with joy. I spent over an hour with Theo laying on my chest, listening to my heart beat. From the moment he was out Jonathan whipped out his camera and was snapping away. He took the most beautiful photo of Theo on my chest, his eyes wide open looking at us both. It was the picture we would send to all of our friends and family to announce his arrival. The picture that would stop hearts beating and fill everyone with so much joy because they had all been on this journey with us.

Before this moment, I still wasn't sure why Gabriel and Raphie didn't make it to be here with us. But when I held Theodore in my arms I instantly knew that he was meant to be here. I knew that this was the baby my soul had longed for, and the baby that would complete our family.

Theodore Louis had arrived and our hearts rejoiced.

## 55

# a church rejoices

Having a baby on Saturday night certainly had its perks. One being the opportunity to surprise everyone with the news at church on Sunday. I asked my mum if she could go to church as normal while Jonathan, Preston and myself spent some time alone with baby Theo.

I wish someone had recorded the moment she stood out the front and shared the news with our church. I'm told it was amazing with so much excitement shared across the room. Mum told them our news and shared Theo's name and the meaning of his name with our church family. Then the photo Jonathan took was put up on the big screen. Everyone was cheering and clapping. Even now it brings a tear to my eye. Our church had become our family. We had shared every part of this journey with them along the way, so to hear how excited they all were made me feel so grateful.

It had been such a long year and our church had backed us in prayer through the heartache and pain, through the good times and the bad. I remember sharing the story of our miscarriages from the front one Sunday. I looked up from my notes to see tissues being passed around and people crying while I shared our story.

When we cried for our babies, they cried too, and when we finally rejoiced over this baby they rejoiced too. Now every week when the worship music plays at church I think back to that moment. I use that time to rejoice and to thank the Lord for all we have and for all that's yet to come.

---

# that's the face

The photo Jonathan took of Theodore the night he was born, holds great spiritual significance for us. I can only imagine the excitement and joy, felt by so many friends and family, when they received that photo, to announce that baby Theo was finally here, safe and sound.

When I sent it to my friend Rebecca she wrote back with three words that I will never forget "That's the face!" She said "Mish! That's the face, that's the baby the Lord showed me with the rings of fire."

My heart felt tight and tears filled my eyes. There are no words to explain how happy I was to hear this. The vision had come full circle. The Lord had fought that spiritual battle for this baby and he was finally here with us, ready to fulfil the plans God had for him. Theodore Louis had arrived and just like in utero, nothing was going to stop him. My little warrior, a gift from God, was here and I would spend the rest of my life thanking the Lord for this journey and the joy we were feeling.

I know for many reading this book your day of rejoicing hasn't come yet. The joy might still seem so far away, or out of reach. My story has a happy ending and I truly believe in my heart that yours will too. The Lord loves you so much and only wants the best for His children. He wants to fulfil all of your hearts desires.

Delight yourself in the Lord and He will give you the desires of your heart (Psalm 37:4).

## *57*

---

# theo

Every mum knows how special and precious her child is. I know that there are so many reasons why each baby or child holds a special place in our hearts. Theo was such a miracle to me. From the moment we found out we were pregnant in hospital and he survived that operation, I knew he was special. In fact, he was a miracle before that, from the moment he was conceived.

Those newborn weeks and the first few months of his life went by so quickly. I made sure to get in as many cuddles as I could and I held on to him so tight. We had a lot of issues in those first few months including a tongue-tie operation and an ongoing case of ductal thrush and mastitis. But no matter what was happening I remained grateful and thankful that he was here. The sleepless nights were worth it. The messy house and the four-year-old competing for our attention, were all worth it. Seeing our beautiful family embrace this little baby and successfully morph into a tribe of four made me feel so happy and so blessed.

Preston was so in love with his baby brother. He asked to hold him every chance he could. He read him stories and sang songs to him. He would sit on the lounge or on his bed and cuddle him for hours. It filled my heart with joy. My family was complete and my heart was full. I became so emotional so many times thinking that this was our miracle, the one we had waited for and prayed for. I was also aware that this was probably the last time I would ever hold my own newborn in my arms. I couldn't take my eyes off him. He was such a sweetheart. Even before he was born we had been through so much together. We share such a special bond and I can feel this fierce connection of love between us.

As Theo grew bigger his smile became his trademark. So cute, so happy, so amazing. You could see so much love in his eyes. His face lit up every time one of us walked in the room (especially his brother). He is my little warrior, and he eats like a warrior too. He's always at the dining table eating, or standing at the fridge asking for more.

When we dedicated Theo at our church we really felt the Lord speaking to us about the Godparents we chose. My brother Michael who loves Preston and Theo so much came to mind. Uncle Mike is certainly a favourite around here and he has a very special bond with both of our boys. Our choice to have him as Godparent came from a much deeper place though. We knew how blessed we were by Theo and we know what a blessing Theo will be to everyone in his life.

The Lord has revealed to us that Theo will play a significant role in Uncle Mike's life and we are so excited for that. Our little boy is already such a wonderful testament to the love of God and the miracles available to us as believers. Theo's Godmother Angela also holds a special place in our hearts and is waiting on her own promise from the Lord. She prayed constantly for Theo during my pregnancy and I can see the love she has for him is like no other. When the Lord put her on my heart to be Theo's Godmother I knew straight away He was uplifting her with hope, hope for her own future promise.

Our little guy is already impacting so many. One Sunday, when he was about 16 months old, we walked into church and he went straight up to our pastor and gave him a hug. This hug was so anointed. Pastor Paul squatted down to greet him and Theo quietly held on tight for about five minutes. Our pastor later revealed that he'd had such a hard week and needed that hug more than we could ever know. Our little boy carries the love of God with him wherever he goes.

I have always felt so strongly that Theo was meant to be here and I know that God has amazing plans for him and his future. It's hard to imagine when you are mourning the loss of a baby that one day you will hold another child against your chest and feel peace in your heart that what happened, was meant to be. It doesn't mean that you love the child you lost any less, but I distinctly remember the moment that I looked into Theo's eyes and it made much more sense. I remembered what my friend Julia told me about Isabel not being here if her first baby had survived. If Gabriel or Raphie had made it into my arms, then Theo wouldn't be here today, and I couldn't imagine this world without him.

I have no idea why the timing of his birth was so important. I have no idea what path this amazing little boy has set before him, but I do know that God's timing is perfect. I can't imagine life without this beautiful boy of mine, that's for sure.

There were times after losing Gabriel that I didn't want another baby to replace him, but Theo isn't a replacement. He is just meant to be here. Gabriel and Raphie each hold a special place in my heart and in our family, just like Preston and Theo do.

For the rest of his life Theo will always remind me that God is good and that no matter what we face or how hard things get, joy always comes in the morning. He reminds me how strong I am, and how fierce a mother's love can be. I hope that at whatever stage of this journey you are in, that God would reveal this to you, and show you how strong you are with Him by your side. I pray that right now He shows you a picture of your future, so you can see that one day you will rejoice again, just like I have.

## 58

a letter to my babies

Gabriel Luca and Raphie Jay,

I want you to know how much I love you. I want you to know that I would give the world just to hold you in my arms. From the moment I knew you were with me I fell deeply in love with you, and nothing will ever change that love. You will always hold a special place in my heart. You are such an important part of our family and I will talk about you and celebrate you all the days of my life.

I'm sorry that things happened this way. I'm sorry that I didn't get to say a proper goodbye, or bury you with the dignity you deserved. But I have to trust that there was a reason for everything that happened. I have to trust that God has a purpose for you in His big picture and that one day I will understand. God knows why we didn't get to meet. He knows why Theodore was meant to be here. When I look into your baby brother's eyes I can't imagine life without him. I'm sure that the day I finally get to look into your eyes, I will feel the same way.

Daddy says hi. I know you mean the world to him too. He's such an amazing dad. I know if you had been given the chance to meet him you would have loved him so much, just like your brothers do. You guys have a lot of wrestling to catch up on when you finally meet. What a beautiful day that will be.

I often wonder what life would be like if you guys were both here with Preston and Theo. I'm sure they would love you just as much as they love each other. One day we will all be together again. That's a promise. Until then, I know that you are safe and loved and looked after. Your time here was short but I promise I loved you for every second of it, and I'll love you for every second of my life too.

I know that our lives here on earth can't compare to your life in heaven. I know that one day I will be there, and I will hold you close, in my arms. I am excited for that day, when I get to see you both.

Please meet me at the gates.

My heart aches for you, my sweet babies.

Love mummy x

## *59*

# a chapter for the dads

You may be reading this book because you are struggling with your own grief, or because you want to better understand what your partner is going through, and the depth of her grief. Maybe your partner has handed you this chapter to read, and I'm so glad she did.

It's important to know that no matter what level of grief or loss you feel, it's ok. It's ok not to understand why your partner is so upset, just as much as it's ok to be totally devastated, heartbroken and shocked to your core.

When we lost our babies, my husband Jonathan was my rock. He held it together, took a week off work to cook and clean and take care of our two-year-old. Not just because of the physical pain I was in, but because he knew I needed him around. There were times I would just start crying all of a sudden and wouldn't be able to stop. I needed him there for those times especially.

Everyone is different, but don't feel pressure to say the right thing or to say too much at all. Most of the time I just needed to cry into Jonathan's arms. I didn't need him to say anything unless he needed to.

If you want to say something but don't know what to say you could simply tell her you love her. Tell her you are always here for her. Tell her you will get through this together. God made you a team for a reason, and so you could be there for each other, for as long as it takes.

People kept telling me "dads are important too!" "dads feel the pain too!" And I totally get that. I often asked Jonathan if he was ok. But I can understand how some mums could be so devastated, that they can't see through the fog, and might not have the energy to check on their partner to see if he's ok. If this is the case for you please don't be disheartened. Sometimes a girl just needs time. The best thing you can do (aside from pray for her), is to tell her you love her and that she should take all the time she needs.

Jonathan told me he was sad when we lost our babies, but mostly he was sad to see me so sad. Even with our first baby, he didn't start getting excited until he could see the bump and feel the baby moving. That's when things felt more real for him, and I can understand that. I felt my baby inside me, and all the changes that come with that, from the moment I knew he was in there. So when I miscarried it's understandable for me to feel the grief a bit deeper than Jonathan did.

If this is the case for you, and your partner is not dealing with the pain as well as you are, that's totally ok and quite normal. As long as you are there for her and supporting her, you are being the best partner to her, and the best dad to your baby already.

Your partner needs love and time. Tell her it's ok to be sad today, happy tomorrow and devastated again the day after. There are no rules, and how you both get through this traumatic ordeal will only make you stronger. It will build your character and you will live to fight another day. Some take longer than others to get through it. Some may never feel "whole" again, like something is missing.

If that's you or your partner it's important to remember that your baby will always be part of your family. They may not be here with you on earth, but that doesn't mean they don't exist. Your baby got an express ticket to heaven. He or she bypassed the pain, suffering, stress and anxiety that fills this world today. Your baby is waiting for you and knows who you are.

If you are a dad who is struggling with his grief then I say give yourself permission to feel the pain. Choose a few mates to talk to, even by a text message to get some support. Cry when you need to cry and tell your partner how you feel. You might be like Jonathan, holding it all together, being a rock for your family, but it's also good to share your pain and grief with your partner. That will bring you closer. It will help her to know how you feel, and it will help you to grieve if you can share your heart with her.

Don't for a second think your pain will be a burden to her. You are just showing her that you are in this together. You are helping to validate her grief, because she's probably worried that the rest of the world won't understand why she's so sad.

An important thing for us on this journey has been that we are honest with each other, and that we always know where we stand with each other. Jonathan and I have been through so many tough times together, and with the help of our faith have managed to come out the other side a much stronger couple because of it.

Jonathan showed his love during this time through actions rather than too many words, and that meant just as much to me. He knew when to pick up a frypan, just like he knew when to sit and be still with me. Sometimes a girl just wants the man she loves to sit next to her for a while, so she doesn't feel alone.

I can't tell you how much it meant to me just for him to be there. Comfort isn't always given in words. If you find it hard to talk about it, then just share some silent moments with her. Hug for as long as it takes and don't say a word. Heat a hot water bottle up for her, make her a cup of tea and just sit with her. Watch as much television as she needs, and let her hold the remote.

Make sure you take time to feel the pain yourself too. You are a dad and you lost your sweet baby. That's significant. That means something. You are allowed to be devastated and you are allowed to cry. You both need to take all the time you need to get through this.

Be there for each other, no matter how long it takes, just be there.

## 60

---

# my soul waits

When I first started writing this book, I had no idea what I was going to call it. How could I put all of this emotion and heartache and hope into the perfect title. I wanted something that would speak to all of the women who had been through what I had, and were looking for hope. I was reading back over my first draft when one of the bible verses God gave me jumped off the page – *I wait for the Lord, my soul waits and in His word I put my hope.*

*My Soul Waits* – I instantly knew that this was the title. When I think of that night, and how I felt when I walked out of the hospital without my baby in my belly or in my arms, the sadness was so much deeper than anything I had ever felt before. It wasn't just my heart that ached but my soul was aching for my baby and it was waiting on that promise.

If you feel that aching deep within your soul, then be assured that you are not alone. The Lord is close to the broken-hearted and saves those who are crushed in spirit. He knows exactly how you feel. He feels it too, and He wants you to feel that joy in your heart, that you so desperately long for.

As I was adding the final touches to this book my friend Philomena sent me a video of a Pastor in the United States named Shawn Bolz. He is a modern day prophet and gave a word of knowledge to a couple who had lost their baby. He stood at the front of a large auditorium and was able to tell this couple, who he had never met before, their names, street name and the names of their children, one child who had passed away.

The couple were emotional and appeared so amazed that God was speaking to them through this pastor. He told them their daughter's name in heaven and said it was never God's intention for her to die, but He was with them the whole way through that time. He saw their little girl in heaven fully formed as God intended.

Things like this strengthen my faith and my hope. There are so many things out there like this that we can find and learn from, that can build our faith. I know where my children are and that our time on earth is so short compared to the eternity that I get to spend with them in heaven.

I've tried so hard to make sure my words in this book have been words of hope, love and faith. I wanted so desperately for every woman reading this to know that there is hope, and that no matter what you have been through, or are going through, you are enough. With God by your side you are strong enough, brave enough, resilient enough, and amazing enough to keep moving forward one minute, one hour, one day at a time.

I hope that this book can be part of your healing journey and give you some peace and reassurance that your baby is safe and loved and that God has the best plans ahead for your family. I hope that from this moment you can allow yourself time to grieve and heal before starting your next chapter.

As I write this final chapter Theo is 18 months old and the sweetest, most beautiful little boy. He gives hope to all of my friends who are waiting on a baby, especially those who have lost a child along the way. I can write this chapter with a heart full of joy and trust in God that He always had the best to come for me and my family. It doesn't mean that I don't still feel that sting when I miss my babies. My soul still waits – maybe not for another baby here on earth but it waits to see Gabriel and Raphie and to hold them in my arms.

I know that some of you have had to wait a lot longer than I have for your heart's desire. I know that some have waited years, and suffered many many more losses than our family. My prayer for you is that God continues to give you strength and hope. I pray you feel His arms wrapped around you. I pray that you feel that He is by your side through it all, and that one day you will be together with your sweet babies again. Ask Him to show you the happy ending that you long for, and then trust Him that it will come, and that it will be everything you ever dreamed of and more.

Until then please reach out for help. You don't need to go through anything alone. There's no need to hide what you are going through or to go through it in secret. Whether it's a local church or support group or counselling that your doctor can recommend please take all the help that you can get. We were put on this earth to help, love and support each other, and getting through something so heartbreaking is much easier with other people on your side.

My mum always tells me that I am braver than I believe, stronger than I seem and smarter than I think, and that I can do all things through Christ who strengthens me. I am declaring this for each and every one of you today. Keep on being brave mumma. There is something inside of you that is stronger than you could ever imagine, you just have to let go, and trust in God that He is with you, and that with Him you are more than enough.

# prayers

I wanted to include some prayers, to help you find that same peace in your heart that I have found when I think about my babies. The first is a short and simple prayer you can pray anytime you're missing your baby, asking for God's comfort and strength. The second is a prayer that we can all say, to ensure our place in heaven next to our babies one day.

*Prayer for the broken-hearted:*

Lord, my heart is aching. I come before you now and ask for your peace and comfort as I mourn the loss of my beautiful baby. There are times that I don't think I can get through this Lord but please give me strength. Help me to feel your loving embrace and to trust you that everything will be ok. Jesus if you could please give my baby a hug for me. Tell them I love them so much and that I miss them every day. Tell them that one day we will be together again. Lord help me to trust you with my child. Help me to keep on living my best life and to feel your love, comfort and protection around me every single day. I pray a blessing over my womb Lord and I pray that you will heal anything related to my womb in the name of Jesus. Lord show me what the future looks like, show me that joy always comes in the morning. Show me that you can turn my mourning into dancing and my sorrow into joy. Thank you Jesus. Thank you for my beautiful baby and the angels surrounding them. In Jesus name I pray, Amen.

*Prayer for our place in heaven:*

Dear Lord, I humble myself before you today. I want to thank you for hearing my prayers and for standing beside me through all the good and the bad in my life. Thank you for always loving me and forgiving me. Lord as my baby resides with you in heaven I want to get to know you better. I want to hear your voice and feel your loving embrace. Lord help me to return to what is most important in this world. Help me to find the love and purpose and direction you have chosen for me. I dedicate my life to you Lord and pray that I too will be in heaven one day with you and my beautiful baby. I invite you into my life and my heart Lord Jesus. Help me on this journey to focus on you, and to grow in your love and strength each day. Thank you Lord, In Jesus name I pray, Amen.

## 62

---

# when God speaks - words of hope

In this final chapter I have included some bible verses which have helped me through my journey, that I thought might help you too. These are such powerful words of hope. Hope for the broken hearted, hope for the weary, hope for the weak, hope for those who love God. It's so hard to find this kind of hope anywhere else in the world. If we find our hope in God then we will never be let down.

All through the bible, God speaks life, love and hope. These verses carried me through the darkest days of my life. I hope and pray that they will speak to you today.

The Lord is close to the brokenhearted and saves those who are crushed in spirit (Psalm 34:18).

Do not fear, for I have redeemed you; I have summoned you by name; you are mine. When you pass through the waters, I will be with you; and when you pass through the rivers, they will not sweep over you. When you walk through fire you will not be burned, and the flames shall not consume you (Isaiah 43:1-2).

My flesh and my heart may fail, but God is the strength of my heart and my portion forever (Psalm 73:26).

When I am afraid, I put my trust in you (Psalm 56:3).

From the ends of the earth I call to you, I call as my heart grows faint; lead me to the rock that is higher than I (Psalm 61:2).

Weeping may stay for the night, but rejoicing comes in the morning (Psalm 30:5).

Be strong and courageous. Do not be frightened, and do not be dismayed, for the Lord your God is with you wherever you go (Joshua 1:9).

When I said, "My foot is slipping," your unfailing love, Lord, supported me. When anxiety was great within me, your consolation brought me joy (Psalm 94:18-19).

God is our refuge and strength, a very present help in trouble. Therefore we will not fear though the earth gives way, though the mountains fall into the heart of the sea, though its waters roar and foam, though the mountains quake with their surging (Psalm 46:1-3).

Cast all your cares on the Lord and he will sustain you (Psalm 55:22).

Whoever dwells in the shelter of the Most High will rest in the shadow of the Almighty. I will say of the Lord, "He is my refuge and my fortress, my God, in whom I trust (Psalm 91:1-2).

I lift up my eyes to the mountains— where does my help come from? My help comes from the Lord, the Maker of heaven and earth. He will not let your foot slip— he who watches over you will not slumber (Psalm 121:1-3).

You will keep in perfect peace those whose minds are steadfast because they trust you (Isaiah 26:3).

"For I know the plans I have for you," declares the Lord, "plans to prosper you and not to harm you, plans to give you hope and a future" (Jeremiah 29:11).

"Because of the Lord's great love we are not consumed, for His compassions never fail" (Lamentations 3:22).

Peace I leave with you, my peace I give to you; not as the world gives do I give to you. Let not your heart be troubled, neither let it be afraid" (John 14:27).

"I consider that our present sufferings are not worth comparing with the glory that will be revealed to us" (Romans 8:18).

"My grace is sufficient for you, for my power is made perfect in weakness" (2 Corinthians 12:9).

Come to me all who are weary and burdened and I will give you rest. Take my yoke upon you and learn from me, for I am gentle and humble in heart, and you will find rest for your souls (Matthew 11:28-30).

Do not fear, for I am with you; do not be dismayed, for I am your God. I will strengthen you and help you; I will uphold you (Isaiah 41:10).

"Do not be anxious about anything, but in every situation, by prayer and petition, with thanksgiving, present your requests to God. And the peace of God, which transcends all understanding, will guard your hearts and your minds in Christ Jesus" (Philippians 4:6-7).

"Whatever is true, whatever is noble, whatever is right, whatever is pure, whatever is lovely, whatever is admirable—if anything is excellent or praiseworthy—think about such things" (Philippians 4:8).

"I can do all things through Him who gives me strength" (Philippians 4:13).

"But the Lord stood at my side and gave me strength" (2 Timothy 4:17).

The Lord is my shepherd; I lack nothing. He makes me lie down in green pastures, he leads me beside quiet waters, he refreshes my soul. He guides me along the right paths for his name's sake. Even though I walk through the darkest valley, I will fear no evil, for you are with me (Psalm 23:1-4).

"There is no fear in love, but perfect love drives out fear" (1 John 4:18)

And we know that in all things God works for the good of those who love him, who have been called according to his purpose (Romans 8:28).

## 63

## thank you

To my beautiful mum (aka Grandma Julz), who continuously drops everything and comes to my rescue. I love you so much. Thank you for your endless love and support of me and my boys. This book and my heart wouldn't be complete without you.

To my dad, who always made me feel like I could do anything if I had my heart and mind in the right place, and for teaching me to fight like Rocky Balboa.

To Mike, whose love as a little brother made me courageous enough, after every fall, to get back up and try again.

To all of our amazing friends, there are so many who weren't mentioned in this book, but we are so grateful for all of your love and support. Thank you for the cards, gifts, flowers, vegetable boxes and precious jewellery, for the advice and encouragement. Thank you for loving our family the way you do. We are forever grateful for each and every one of you.

To Pastor Paul and our church family at Lifehouse Church. What would we have done without you backing us in prayer, your spiritual wisdom, your endless love and your home-cooked meals? We are so blessed by you guys every single day and we can feel God's love for us through each and every one of you (especially my sisters in Christ).

To the beauties who read this book before I was brave enough to share it with the world. Iliana, Tracey, Natalie, Philomena, Evelyne, Jenny and mum. I am so grateful for you all. Thank you for giving me the confidence to share my story.

To our families: our mums and dads, nanna, our brothers and sisters and extended families who loved and supported us unconditionally through it all, what a blessing you all are. To my beautiful cousins: Belinda, who inspired me to write this book, you constantly show me the true meaning of brave; and to Karen for those beautiful olive trees. I love you both so much.

To Jonathan and my beautiful boys Preston and Theodore, my heart is full because of you. You made me a mum and taught me how to love without limits. You are my world, and I am who I am because of you.

To Gabriel and Raphie, thank you for showing me a new depth of love, and helping me to trust in something much bigger than myself. I wish I could hold you in my arms, just once. My heart aches for you both. I hope you will always know how much I love you.

And finally to the one and only, my Lord and Saviour, Jesus Christ. My heart and soul rejoice and it's all because of you.

# appendix

*Jesse: found in heaven*
Author: Chris Pringle
Publication date: April, 2005
Publisher: Whitaker House

*Heaven Is for Real*
Author: Todd Burpo and Lynn Vincent
Publication date: November 2, 2010
Publisher: Nelson

*The Beautiful Truth*
Author: Mark Anthony
Publication Date: 10 August 2016
Publisher: Createspace Independent Pub (10 August 2016)

www.ingramcontent.com/pod-product-compliance
Lightning Source LLC
Chambersburg PA
CBHW032137020426
42334CB00016B/1197